Surgical Pathological Anatomy of Head and Neck Specimens

Springer
London
Berlin
Heidelberg
New York
Barcelona
Hong Kong
Milan
Paris
Santa Clara
Singapore
Tokyo

P.J. Slootweg and J.A.M. de Groot

Surgical Pathological Anatomy of Head and Neck Specimens

A Manual for the Dissection of Surgical Specimens from the Upper Aerodigestive Tract

With 107 Figures
including 41 in colour

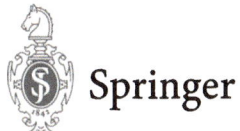

Springer

Pieter J. Slootweg
University Hospital, Department of Pathology, HP 04.314,
P.O. Box 85.500, 3508 GA Utrecht, The Netherlands

John A.M. de Groot
University Hospital, Department of Otorhinolaryngology, HP DO5.244,
P.O. Box 85.500, 3508 GA Utrecht, The Netherlands

British Library Cataloguing in Publication Data
Slootweg, P.J.
    Surgical pathological anatomy of head and neck specimens:
    a manual for the dissection of surgical specimens from the
    upper aerodigestive tract
    1. Human dissection – Handbooks, manuals, etc. 2. Head –
    Dissection – Handbooks, manuals, etc. 3. Neck – Dissection –
    Handbooks, manuals, etc.
    I. Title   II. Groot, J.A.M. de
    611.3

Library of Congress Cataloging-in-Publication Data
Slootweg, Pieter Johannes, 1950–
    Surgical pathological anatomy of head and neck specimens: a
manual for the dissection of surgical specimens from the
upper aerodigestive tract / P.J. Slootweg & J.A.M. de Groot. – 1st ed.
        p.   cm.
    Includes bibliographical references.
    ISBN 978-1-4471-1213-6   ISBN 978-1-4471-0831-3 (eBook)
    DOI 10.1007/978-1-4471-0831-3

    1. Head – Cancer – Diagnosis.   2. Neck – Cancer – Diagnosis.
3. Pathology, Surgical – Technique.   4. Head – Dissection.   5. Neck – Dissection.
6. Pathology, Surgical – Technique.   I. Groot, J.A.M. de, 1947– .   II. Title.
    [DNLM: 1. Head and Neck Neoplasms – pathology.   2. Dissection – methods.
3. Specimen Handling – methods.   4. Pathology, Surgical – methods   WE 707 S634s 1999]
RD661.S63   1999
616.99′491 – dc21
DNLM/DLC   98–43506
for Library of Congress   CIP

Typeset by EXPO Holdings, Malaysia

28/3830-54321 Printed on acid-free paper

Preface

The dissection of surgical specimens from the upper aerodigestive tract is often difficult due to the anatomically complicated nature of this area. Local environment dictates routes of tumour spread and surgical margins at risk and these features differ for various subsites within this part of the body. Moreover, adequate investigation of surgical specimens of the upper aerodigestive tract requires knowledge of the various types of surgical procedures used for different areas and should provide data that enable the surgeon to correlate preoperatively performed diagnostic imaging with the macroscopic findings obtained postoperatively.

The aim of this book is to provide guidelines for the anatomical dissection of specimens from oral and sinonasal cavities, pharynx and larynx. This is done by illustrations that combine drawings of tumours at various anatomical subsites, details of the respective surgical procedures, the specimens thus obtained, and the way to dissect these specimens as shown by colour photographs of surgical specimens handled in the way schematically outlined.

The book will be of benefit for pathologists, oral and maxillofacial surgeons, ENT surgeons and residents in training for these specialties.

Contents

Introduction

Head and Neck Specimens and Surgical Pathology

Optimal patient care requires close cooperation between clinician and pathologist. Of course this statement applies to patient treatment in its widest sense. However, it applies especially to surgical pathology of the head and neck area where surgical specimens are anatomically complicated, containing many different structures and tissue types confined within a limited volume. Most often the surgeon does not require the diagnosis, which is usually known beforehand, but is more interested in knowing which structures are invaded by tumour, whether the margins are free, and whether preoperative diagnostic imaging has given a true picture of tumour size and extension. Examination of surgically resected head and neck specimens is thus a demanding task that requires knowledge of anatomy, types of surgical resections and macroscopic clinicopathological data that are important for assessment of the need for additional treatment postoperatively.

It is the purpose of this book to discuss and illustrate the way in which surgical specimens from the head and neck area should be handled to retrieve the maximum of information that will enable the surgeon to give patients optimal treatment. In this way the surgical pathologist will become, and remain, an esteemed member of the head and neck oncological team.

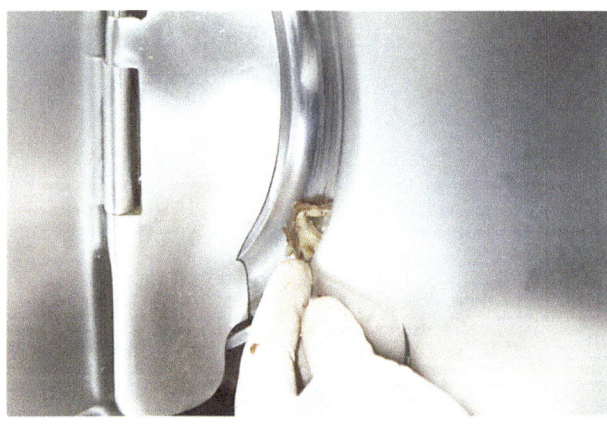

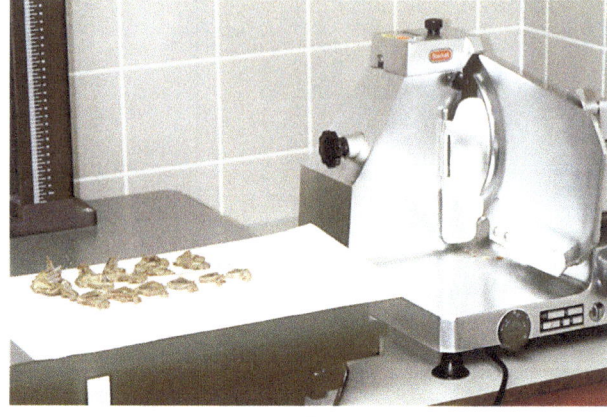

a   b

Figure 1.1 ▲ Slicing device to obtain 4 mm thick slices from laryngeal specimens. By making slices in this way the tumour dimensions and involvement of various laryngeal compartments are easily visualised.

a Positioning of larynx in the apparatus and making slices.

b Positioning of the slices, with the cranial surface above and the ventral surface to the left.

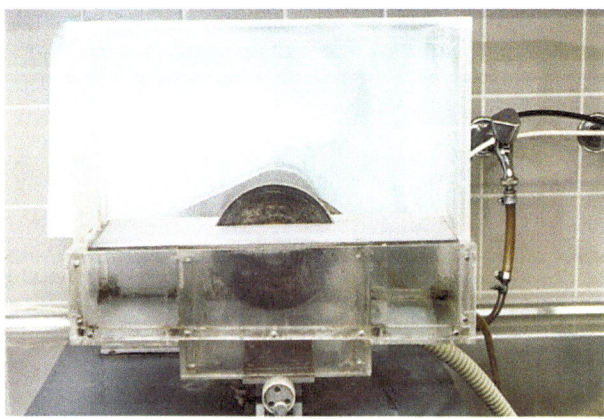

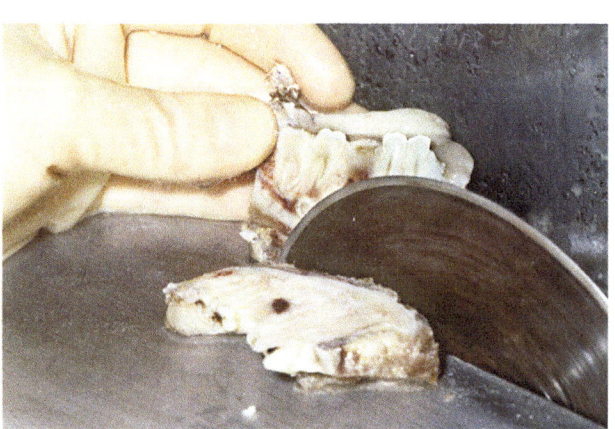

a   b

Figure 1.2 ▲ Engine-driven water-cooled diamond saw to obtain slices from jaw specimens including bone and teeth with, if present, dental artefacts.

a Apparatus consisting of a saw and height-adjustable table encased in a Plexiglas frame.

b By gently pressing the specimen against the blade, slices of a thickness as low as 2 mm can be obtained. As the specimen is sliced by grinding, and not by cutting as would be the case with a toothed saw, soft tissues are not torn away from the bony surface. Therefore, complete slices of the specimen are obtained allowing assessment of tumour dimensions and spread.

General Technical Notes

As the majority of head and neck resections are performed to treat head and neck squamous cell cancer, this tumour will be the example used to discuss the types of surgical specimens obtained from various sites unless explicitly stated otherwise. Before going into detail, however, we will mention some general principles that apply to all kinds of resections.

For any specimen it is mandatory to recognise the anatomical components that are part of it, to note whether it comes from the right or the left side, to measure the size of the mucosal surfaces and to identify, measure and describe mucosal changes (if present). Moreover, one should mention which anatomical structures form the surgical margins and the natural surfaces of the specimen. If a neck dissection is done in continuity with removal of the site of the primary lesion, the neck dissection forming part of the specimen, one should dissect the neck from the primary tumour site through an anatomical plane; this allows easier handling of the part of the specimen that contains the tumour, while the neck can be investigated as a separate specimen.

After cutting the specimen one should measure the thickness of the lesion, the structures that are involved, the resection margin that is closest to the lesion, and the anatomical area of which this closest margin forms a part. Often it is helpful to make photographs or drawings of the specimen and the cut slices that may be used to identify samples taken for histological examination. Standard drawings, diagrams or checklists [1] can also be used for this purpose. Finally, as head and neck specimens often contain mineralised structures such as bone and teeth or, in the case of the larynx, cartilage that may be ossified, technical equipment allowing slicing of these resection specimens should be available. For the larynx, the commercially available slicing machine as introduced by Michaels and Gregor [2] is indispensable (Fig. 1.1). For maxillofacial specimens containing bone and teeth, a water-cooled diamond grinding blade is mandatory (Fig. 1.2). By using these types of apparatus it is possible to make slices without separating the soft tissues from either bone or cartilage and thus to obtain a good cut surface that clearly shows how the tumour involves the relevant anatomical structures. Making a specimen cuttable by immersing it in decalcification solution allows further processing only after a long time and leads to unacceptable loss of macroscopic as well as microscopic features.

Anatomy

Head and neck specimens come from the following anatomical regions: oral cavity, larynx, pharynx and (sino)nasal cavities. As almost all malignancies metastasise to the lymph nodes in the neck, neck dissections of various types are probably the specimens from the head and neck area that are encountered most often. All these anatomical regions can be subdivided, and we will discuss the various types of specimens coming from these sites. For each location we will discuss the anatomical extension, the common type of specimen, the standard method of dissection and, if applicable, other site-specific features.

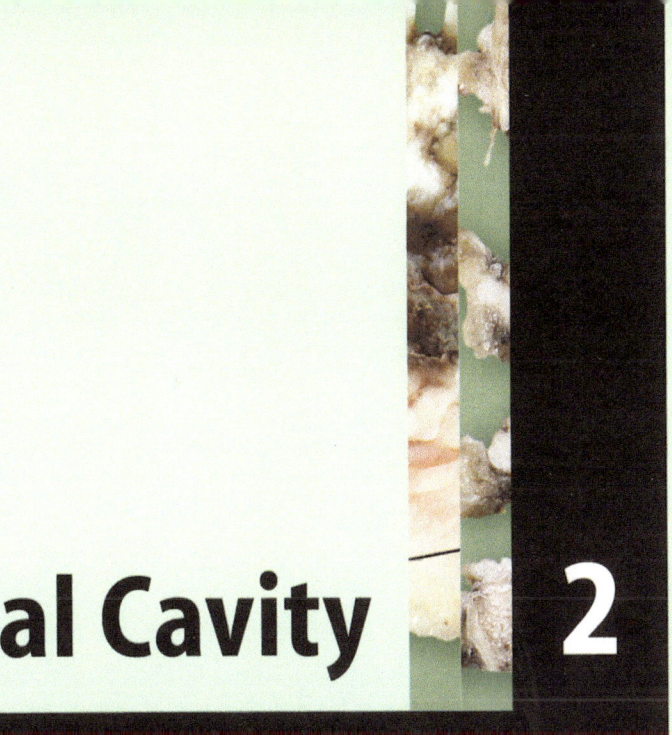

Oral Cavity 2

Anatomical Subregions

Within the oral cavity several anatomical subregions can be discerned: the upper and lower lip, oral vestibule, maxilla, mandible, retromolar trigone, floor of the mouth, tongue, and cheek. Site-specific characteristics and clinicopathological features will be discussed separately for the various locations.

Lip

Anatomy

The lip represents an area that begins at the junction of the vermilion border with the skin. Intraorally the mucosa of the lip merges imperceptibly with the mucosa of the oral vestibule.

Specimen

Most surgical resections from the lower lip are performed to treat squamous cell cancer. Resections from the upper lip are mostly done for submucosally located salivary gland tumours. In both instances the specimen is a wedge-shaped or more rectangular-shaped excision with a muscular core, one side covered by skin, the opposite side covered by mucosa and the vermilion border forming a longitudinal strip at the junction of skin and mucosa at the free edge of the specimen. The mucosa-covered intraoral part of the specimen may contain a part of the oral vestibule, depending on the size and location of the

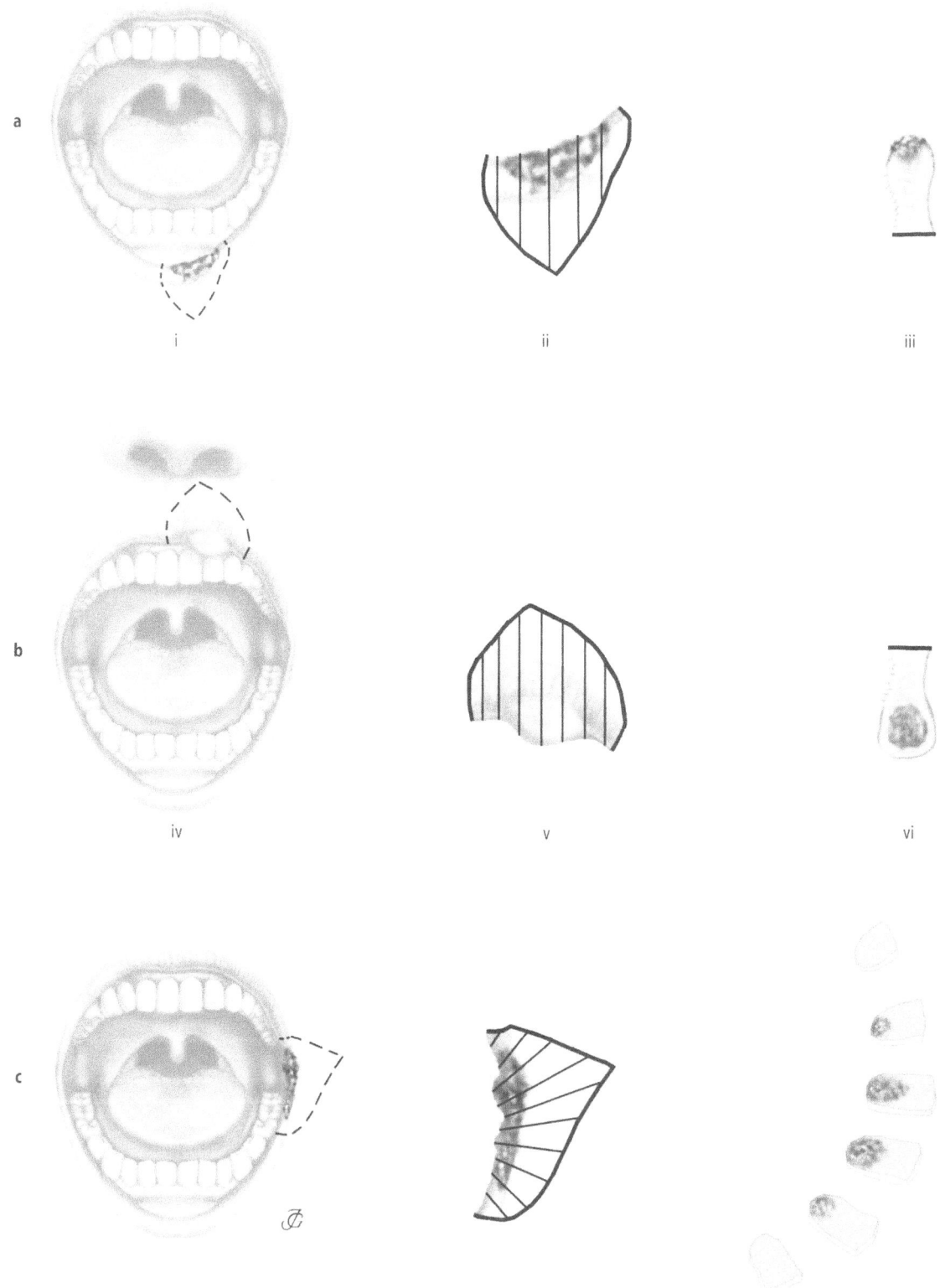

Figure 2.1

lesion. At its left or right lateral side the resection may extend into the corner of the mouth, the area where upper and lower lip and cheek mucosa meet.

Dissection

If the resection is done for treatment of squamous cell cancer, gross examination starts with determining the size and site of the lesion, identifying the area where the lesion lies closest to the surgical margin and measuring the distance between the lesion and this margin. Thereafter, the specimen is cut from left to right perpendicular to the free edge of the lip. In this way, slices are obtained that exhibit a full-thickness view of the lip and the lesion (Fig. 2.1). When the specimen contains squamous cell cancer, the depth of invasion should be measured. When the specimen contains a more deeply seated salivary gland tumour, the maximal size should be recorded as well as its outline, which may be either circumscribed or ill-defined (Fig. 2.2, *page 8*).

Specific Features

If the resection extends into the corner of the mouth, the rules for dissecting cheek specimens apply for this part of the specimen. In practice, this means continuing to make slices perpendicular to the mucosal surface. At the junction between the lip and the corner of the mouth, the mucosal surface exhibits a 90° angle; to follow this angulation it is necessary to make wedge-shaped slices that will exhibit the deep margin through the musculature (Fig. 2.1c).

Oral Vestibule

The oral vestibule is the space between the cheek and the inner side of the upper and lower lip on one side and the maxilla and mandible on the other side. It is a horseshoe-shaped space without clearly defined boundaries, its mucosal surface merging with the mucosal lining of the adjacent structures. This mucosal area may form part of resections done for lesions occurring in these adjacent structures (cancer of lip, cheek or gingiva) that extend into this area of the oral cavity. No specimens are restricted to the oral vestibule as single site.

Maxilla

Anatomy

The maxilla consists of the horseshoe-shaped alveolar ridge that contains the teeth and that encloses the other component of the maxilla, the hard palate. The bony maxilla separates the oral cavity from the nasal cavity and, more dorsally, also from the maxillary sinus. At its oral side the maxillary bone, alveolar ridge as well as hard palate, is covered with a mucosal lining that is firmly attached to the underlying periosteum. In the case of a dentate jaw this mucosal lining is also attached to the dental root areas that protrude from the alveolar sockets; this specialised mucosa is called the gingiva. Laterally and anteriorly the mucosa that covers the maxilla at its oral side merges with the mucosal lining of the oral vestibule. Dorsally the maxilla ends at the junction with the soft palate and the tonsillar pillars,

Dissection of lip resections.

a Cancer of the lower lip. Site of the tumour with the outline of the resection: i, surgical specimen; ii, plane of sectioning; iii, cut surface.

b For the upper lip, the example of a submucous salivary gland lesion is chosen: iv, the submucosal swelling with the outline of the resection; v, the surgical specimen and the plane of sectioning; vi, the cut surface clearly displaying the submucosally located lesion.

c Cancer of the lower lip extending into the left corner of the mouth: vii, the site and extension of the lesion with the outline of the resection; viii, the resected specimen and the plane of sectioning, which is rotating to accommodate the bent median axis of the specimen; ix, the slices thus obtained.

Figure 2.1
◄

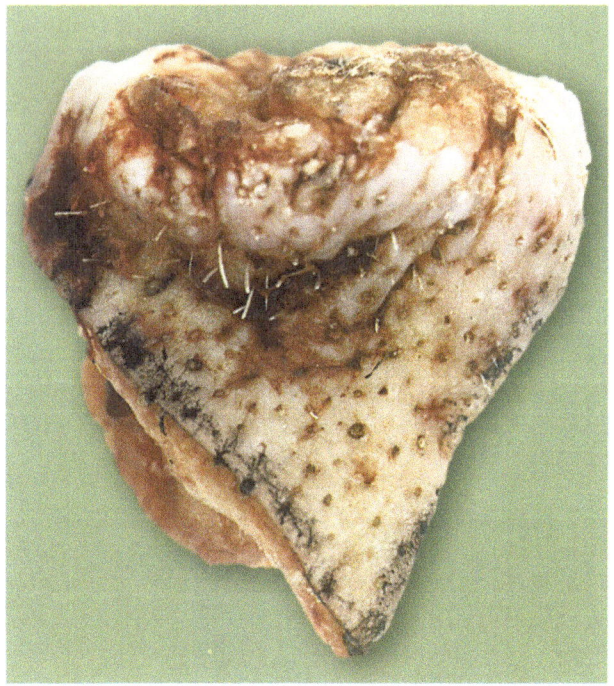

a

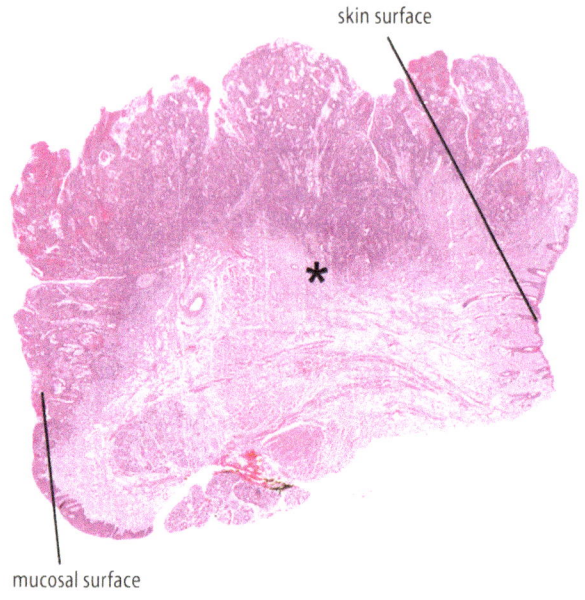

skin surface

mucosal surface

b

skin surface

mucosal surface

c

Figure 2.2
▲

a Lip resection performed to treat squamous cell cancer at the vermilion border.

b Mounted haematoxylin and eosin stained section of squamous cell cancer of the lip displaying skin as well as mucosal surface. The tumour at the vermilion border penetrates into the underlying muscular tissue (*).

c Mounted haematoxylin and eosin stained section of lip resection with submucosally located adenoid cystic carcinoma.

which both belong to the oropharynx. Slightly thickened mucosal pads, the maxillary tuberosities, form the dorsal part of the alveolar ridge. At its cranial side the maxilla is covered by respiratory epithelium that lines the lower surface of the nasal cavity or maxillary sinus.

Specimen

Resections involving the maxilla are usually done for squamous cell cancer of the mucosa of the alveolar ridge or the hard palate. Less often the reason for a partial or complete maxillectomy is a salivary gland tumour occurring submucosally at the hard palate, a sarcoma arising within the maxillary bone, a fibro-osseous lesion, or an intraosseous odontogenic tumour.

A maxillectomy specimen shows an oral surface covered by squamous epithelium that lines the palatal bone as well as the alveolar ridge and that in dentate jaws is connected with the necks of the teeth to form the maxillary gingiva. The opposite side represents the bottom of the nasal cavity and maxillary sinus, from which a vertical bony ridge protrudes representing the lateral nasal wall, splitting dorsally to become the lateral wall of the maxillary sinus and the lateral nasal wall which is also the medial maxillary sinus wall. If a substantial part of the lateral nasal wall forms part of the specimen it includes the lower nasal turbinate, which can be seen protruding from the medial surface of this bony structure. If the resection crosses the midline, the dorsal specimen surface also contains the lower part of the nasal septum. The horizontal margins through these two – or three if the midline is crossed – vertical bony ridges represent the cranial borders of a maxillectomy specimen. The other margins are through the zygomatic bone laterally, the alveolar ridge anteriorly, and the hard palate medially. Posteriorly the resection margin may still go through the hard palate if the lesion is not too large; for more extended lesions, this margin goes through the soft palate. Thus a maxillectomy specimen is a disc with upper and lower natural surfaces, surgical margins lying circumferentially at the periphery of the disc, and crossing the vertical bony ridges that connect the maxilla with the skull base (Fig. 2.3, page 10).

In the case of limited lesions or benign lesions the surgeon may save the palatal bone, only removing the palatal mucosa with submucosa while curetting the underlying bone. In these instances there is also a deep surgical margin (Figs. 2.4, page 11, 2.5, page 12).

Dissection

Before dissecting the specimen one should determine externally visible features. In the case of mucosal lesions one should record their size and site. In the case of centrally located lesions one should notice their location and observe whether they have caused externally visible swelling and whether they perforate through a natural surface, which may be either the nasal or the oral one.

In all cases it is mandatory to dissect the specimen in such a way that parallel slices are obtained. Usually this requires the use of the engine-driven water-cooled diamond saw to cut slices in which bone, teeth with or without dental restorations and soft tissues retain their mutual anatomical relationship. For the posterior parts of the maxilla the plane of sectioning will be frontal. This allows comparison of the slices with CT scans or MRI scans that are made in the same direction and thus evaluation of the preoperatively performed diagnostic imaging (Figs. 2.6, page 12, 2.7, page 13).

For resections that consist of the anterior median part of the maxilla, the plane of sectioning will be sagittal (Figs. 2.8, 2.9, page 14). In the case of resections containing the posterior as well as the anterior part of the maxilla, such as a hemimaxillectomy, one has to follow the parabolic curve of the teeth row and alveolar ridge in cutting slices. This is done as follows: the premolar–molar area of the maxilla is cut in slices parallel to the frontal plane. Thereafter, the remaining part of the specimen is cut in wedge-shaped slices that display the surgical margin facing the oral vestibule. The most median slice will represent the anterior part of the median surgical margin (Fig. 2.10, page 15).

The cut surfaces of the slices will clearly display the extension of the lesion and the structures involved. The following items have to be noted: maximal size of lesion, maximal depth of infiltration in the case of mucosal squamous cell carcinoma, minimal distance to the margin and location of this closest margin, and whether there is penetration of tumour into the nasal cavity, maxillary sinus or periodontal ligament space (Fig. 2.11, page 16). For submucosal lesions one should record whether the

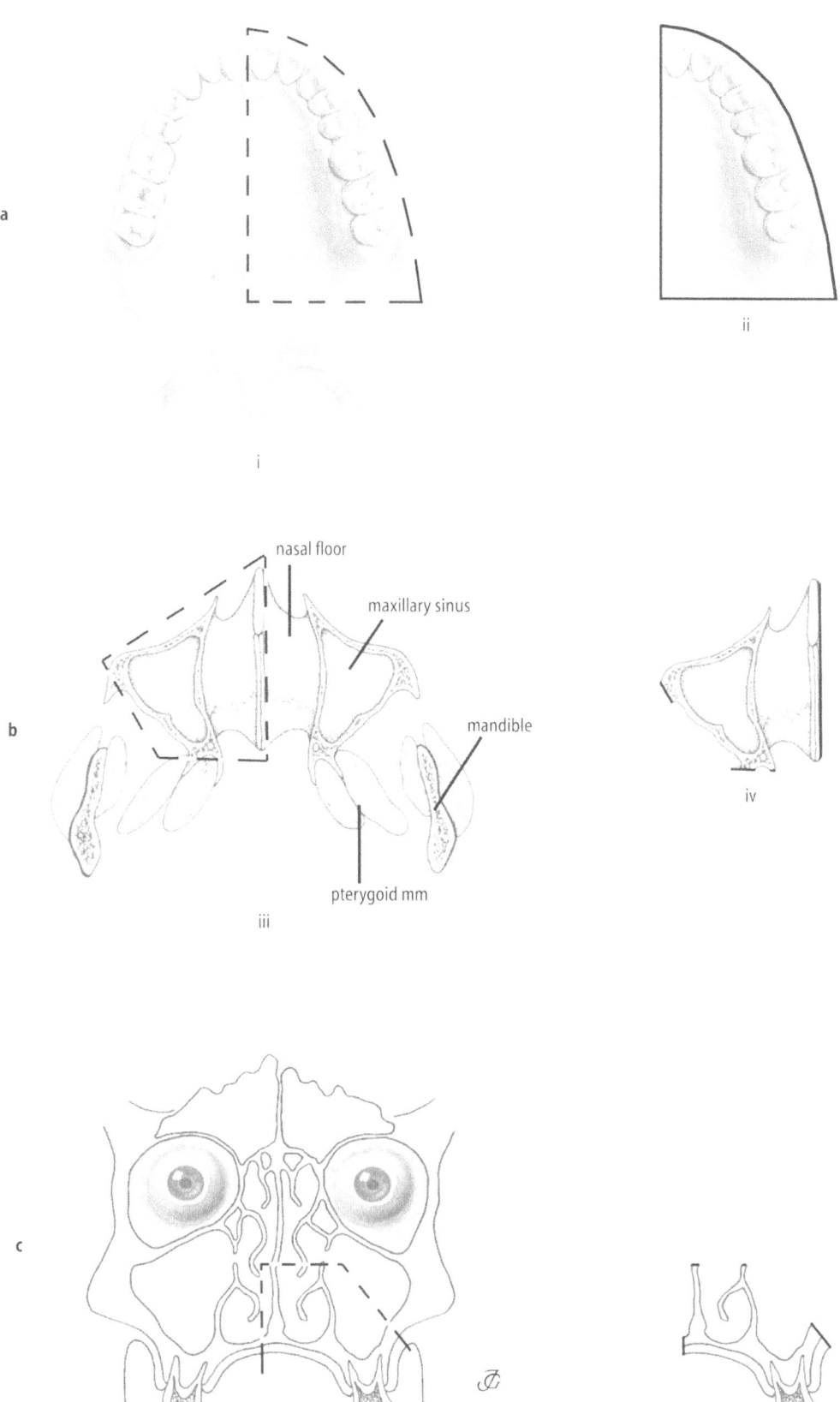

a

i

ii

b

nasal floor

maxillary sinus

mandible

pterygoid mm

iii

iv

c

v

vi

Figure 2.3

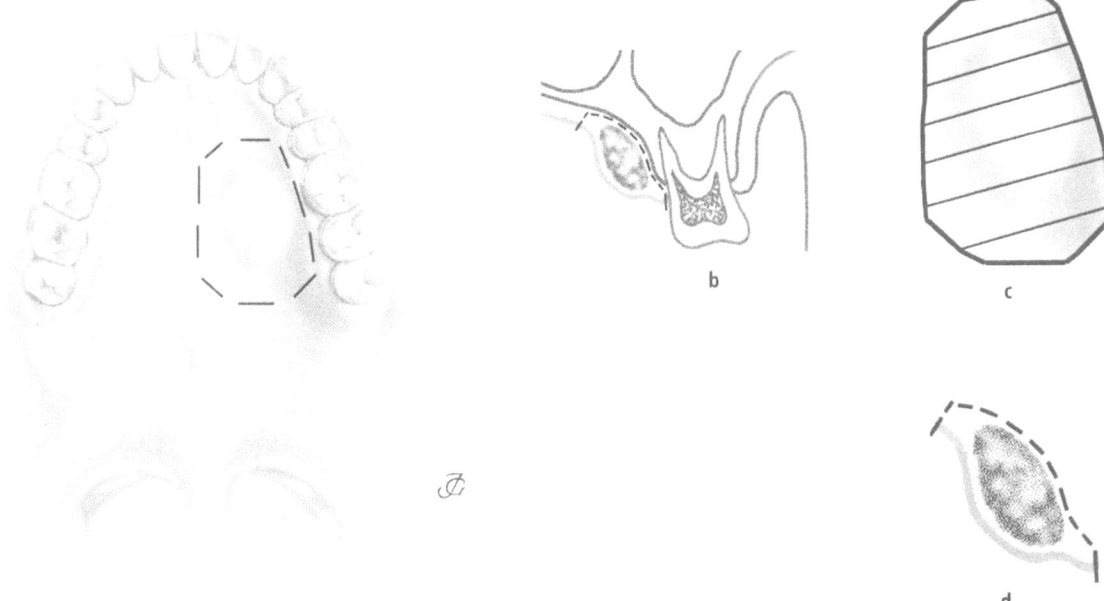

a   d

Pathological anatomy of benign submucosal lesions at the hard palate, e.g. a pleiomorphic
adenoma.

a Clinical appearance with outline of the resection.

b Frontal plane to show tumour with surrounding structures and outline of the resection.

c Surgical specimen and plane of sectioning.

d Cut surface.

Figure 2.4
▲

Pathological anatomy of the maxilla and hard palate.

a Oral surface of the hard and soft palate and teeth row with an outline of the hemimaxillectomy (i) as well as the specimen (ii).

b Cranial surface of the maxilla that consists of the maxillary sinus floor and nasal floor and is
bordered dorsally by the pterygoid process as well as musculature. Extension of the hemimaxillectomy specimen is shown by a dashed line in iii and the specimen itself is shown in iv.
Three bony ridges connect the maxilla with the skull base.

c Frontal view of the maxilla with surrounding structures. The extension of the hemimaxillectomy is depicted by a dashed line in v and shown separately in vi.

Figure 2.3
◄

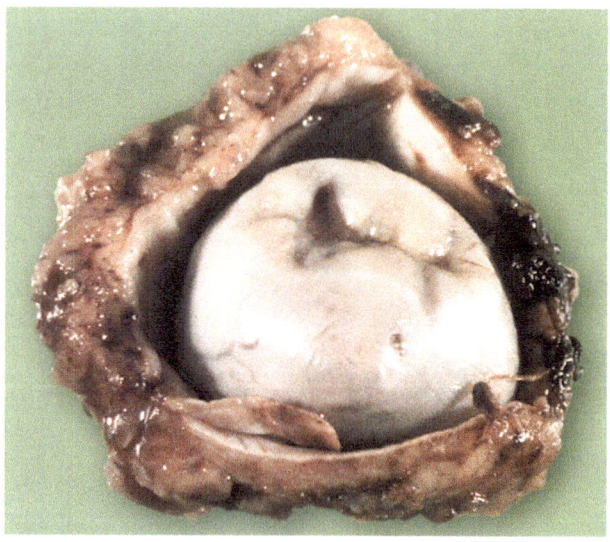

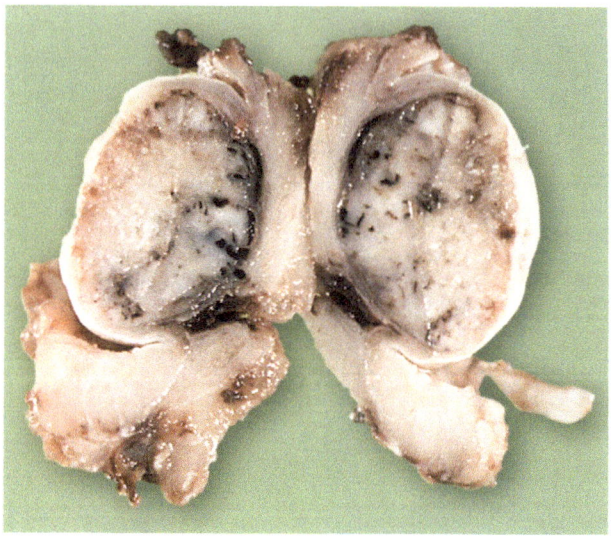

a

b

Figure 2.5
▲

Macroscopic appearance of a surgical specimen with a benign salivary gland lesion of the hard palate.

a Macroscopic appearance.

b Cut surface displaying the circumscribed lesion.

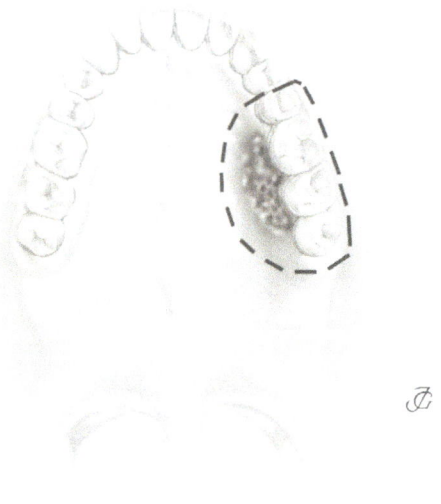

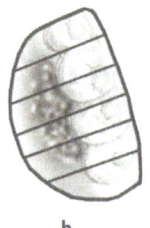

b

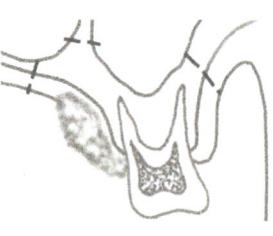

a

c

Figure 2.6
▲

Pathological anatomy of cancer at the palatal gingiva in the posterior part of the maxilla.

a Clinical appearance and outline of the resection.

b Surgical specimen and plane of sectioning.

c Cut surface displaying tumour site and thickness as well as involvement of adjacent structures and outline of the resection.

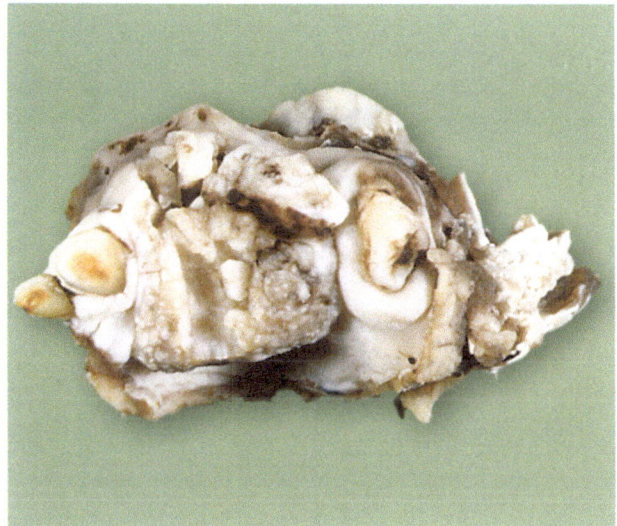

a

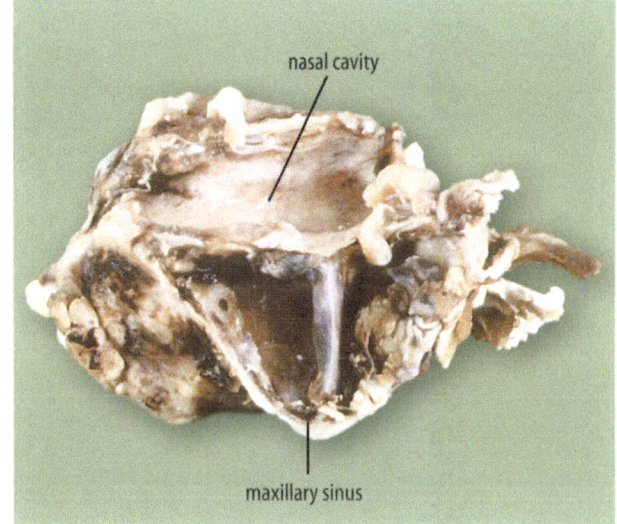

nasal cavity

maxillary sinus

b

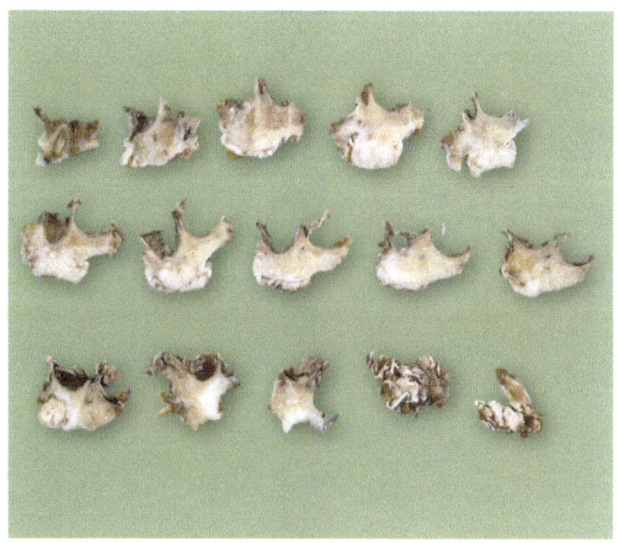

c

Macroscopic appearance of cancer at the alveolar process and hard palate of the maxilla.

a Palatal surface of specimen showing exophytic tumour. Teeth can be seen adjacent to the tumour ventrally as well as dorsally.

b Cranial surface of specimen showing the nasal cavity as well as the floor of the maxillary sinus. The latter shows a bony crest separating the maxillary sinus into an anterior and a posterior part.

c Slices obtained when cutting the specimen buccopalatally.

Figure 2.7
▲

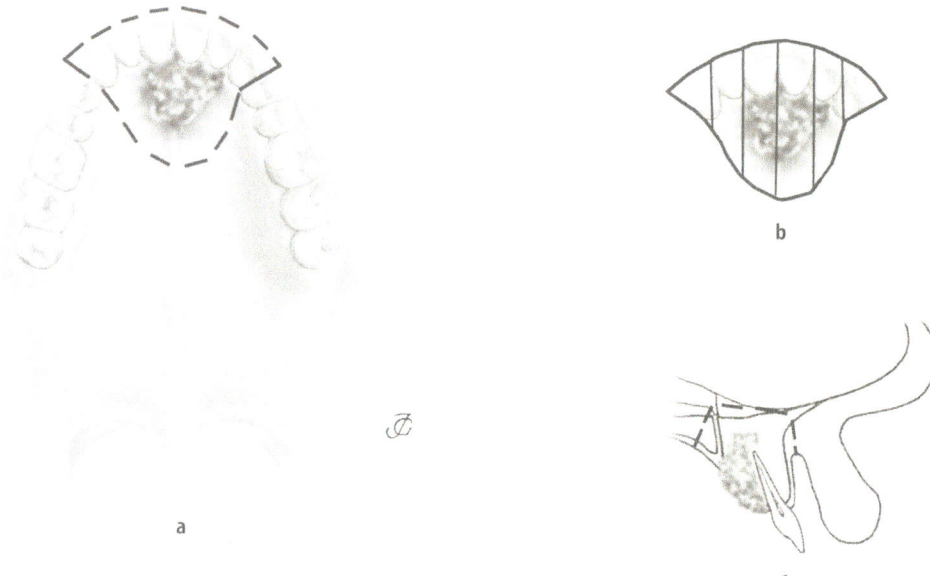

a

b

c

Figure 2.8
▲

Pathological anatomy of gingival cancer in the anterior part of the maxilla.

a Clinical appearance and outline of the resection.

b Surgical specimen and plane of sectioning.

c Cut surface displaying tumour site and thickness as well as involvement of adjacent structures and outline of the resection.

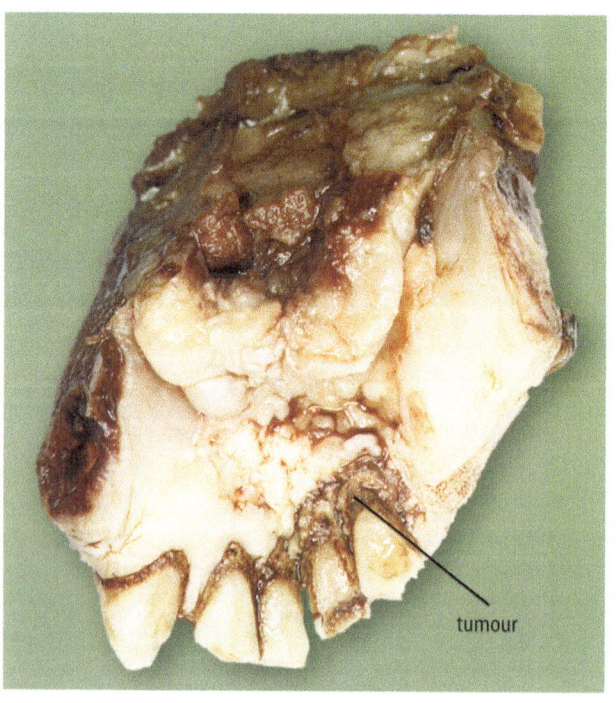

tumour

Figure 2.9
▲

Palatal view of cancer in the anterior maxilla. Tumour can be seen at the gingival margin.

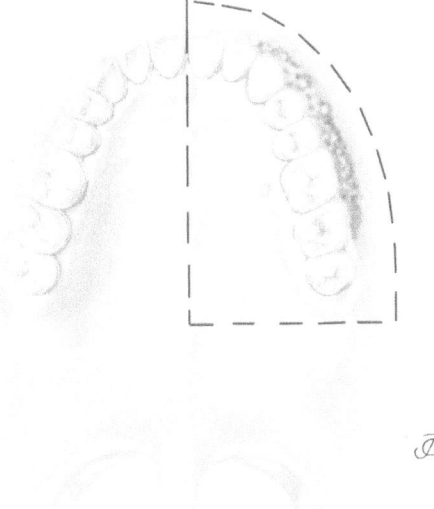

a

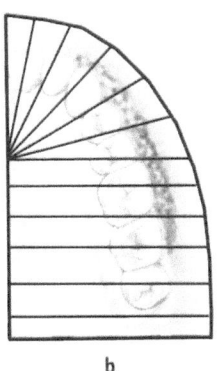

b

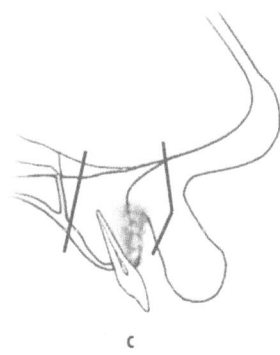

c

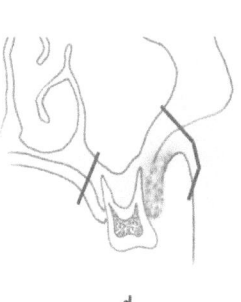

d

Pathological anatomy of buccal gingival cancer involving the entire left upper jaw.

a Tumour extension and outline of the resection.

b Surgical specimen and plane of sectioning, which rotates to accommodate the parabolic curve of the teeth row.

c Cut surface and outline of the resection at the anterior part of the specimen.

d Cut surface and outline of the resection at the posterior part of the specimen.

Figure 2.10
▲

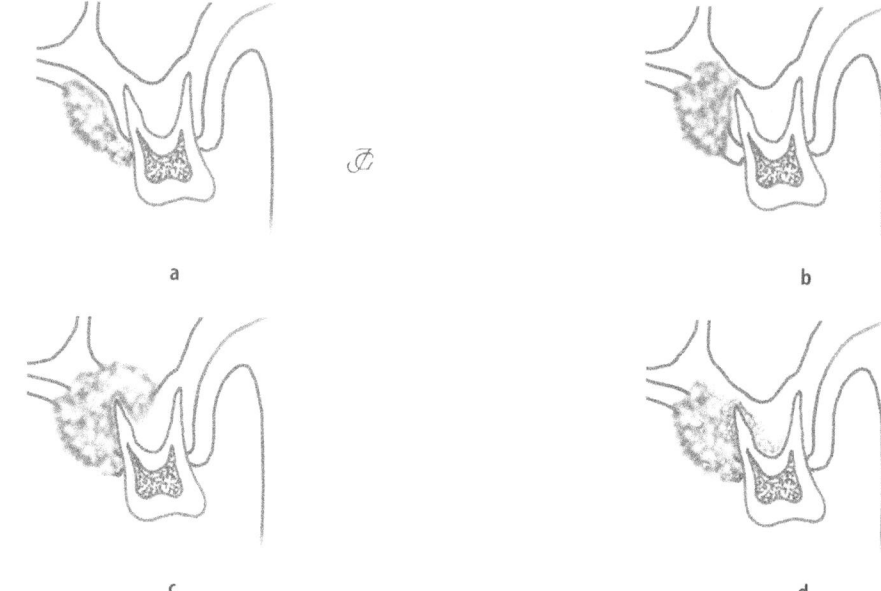

Figure 2.11

Drawings illustrating the various ways in which palatal gingival cancer may spread into adjacent structures.

a Lesion confined to mucosa and submucosa.

b Spread into underlying bone.

c Extension into the maxillary sinus.

d Involvement of the periodontal ligament space of adjacent teeth.

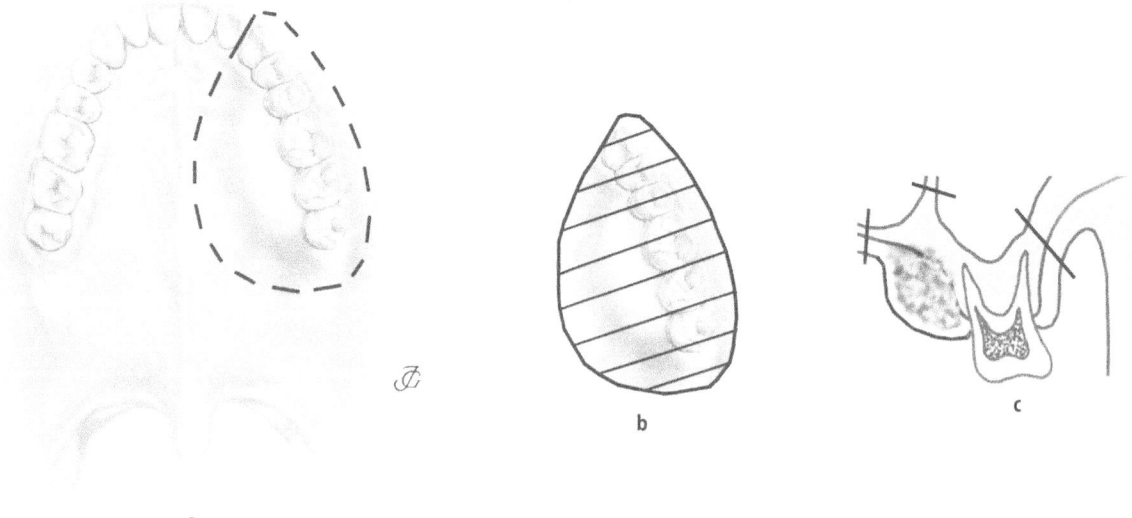

Figure 2.12

Pathological anatomy of a submucosally located lesion at the hard palate.

a Clinical appearance and outline of the resection.

b Surgical specimen and plane of sectioning.

c Cut surface showing tumour extension and outline of the resection. This presentation is characteristic for both benign and malignant salivary gland tumours.

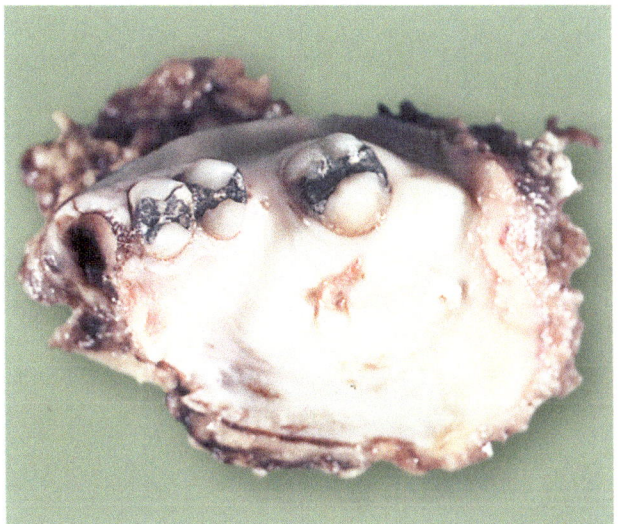

a

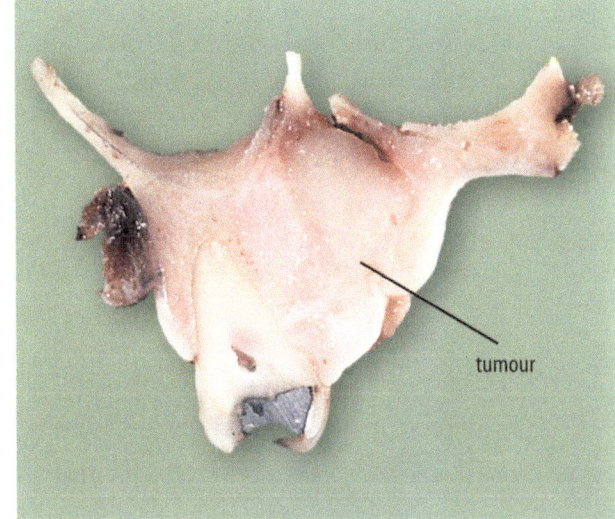

tumour

b

Macroscopic appearance of submucosally located salivary gland tumour at the hard palate.

a Palatal view showing swelling at the palate covered by a mucosal surface with a tiny defect due to previous biopsy.

b Slice obtained by cutting in a buccopalatal direction, displaying tumour destroying adjacent palatal bone.

Figure 2.13
▲

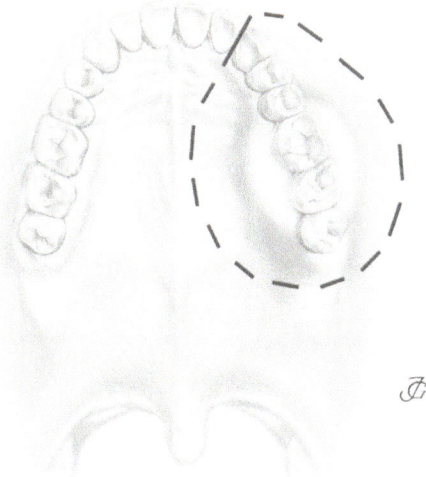

a

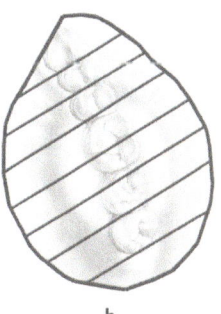

b

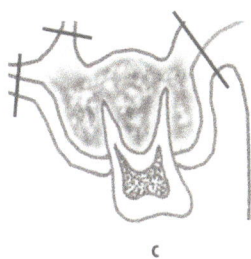

c

Pathological anatomy of intraosseous maxillary tumour.

a Clinical appearance and outline of the resection.

b Surgical specimen and plane of sectioning.

c Cut surface showing tumour extension and outline of the resection. This presentation is typical for lesions of the maxillary bone such as osteosarcoma, ossifying fibroma and odontogenic tumours.

Figure 2.14
▲

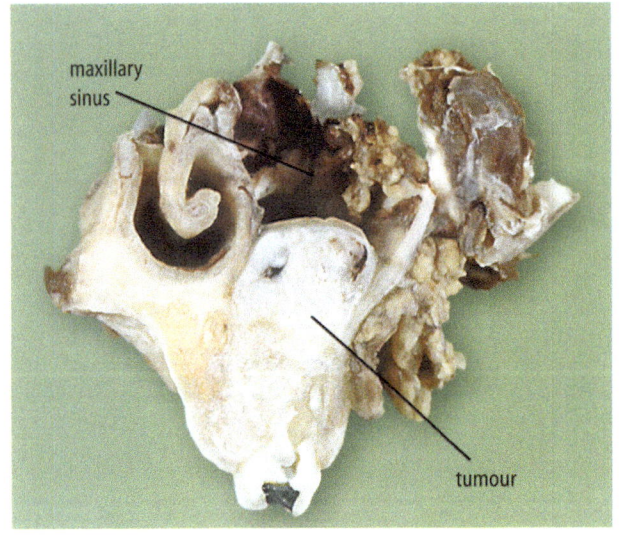

a

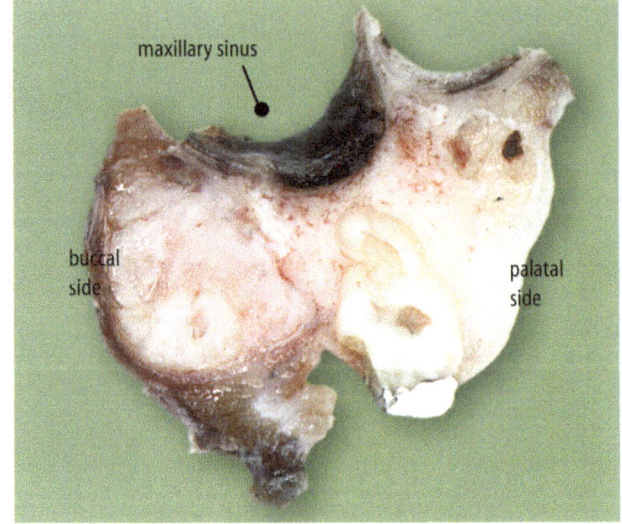

b

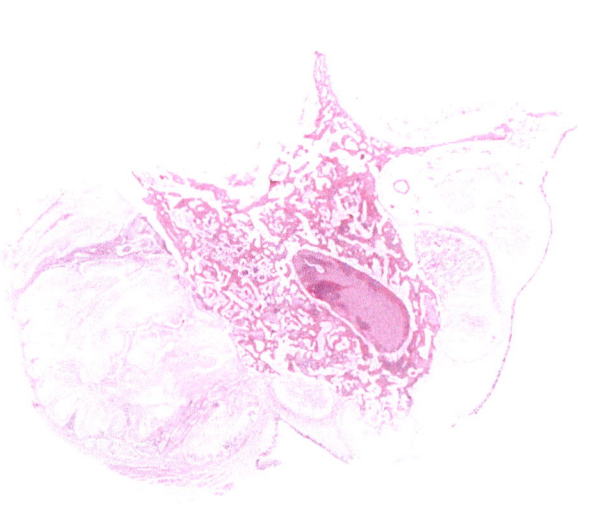

c

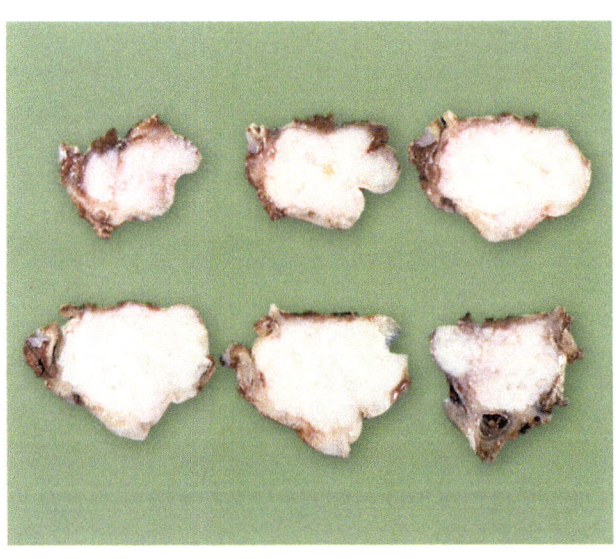

d

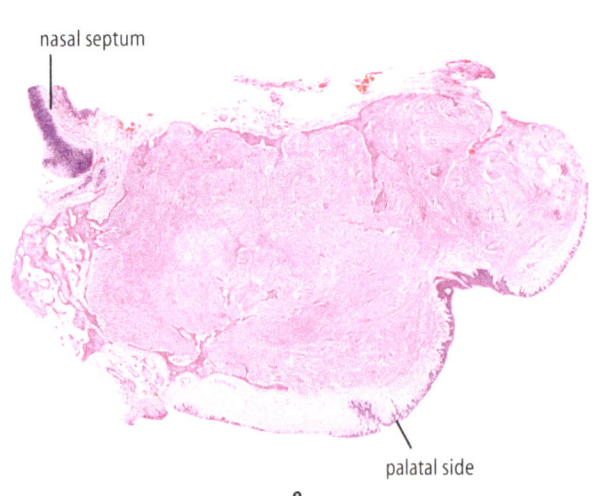

e

Figure 2.15

lesion lies between the mucosal lining of the palate and the underlying palatal bone, as is the case for salivary gland tumours (Figs. 2.12, *page 16*, 2.13, *page 17*), or whether the lesion lies in the maxillary bone. If the lesion is intraosseous one should note whether it remains confined within the bone – with or without expansion and attenuation of the cortical bone – or whether the cortical border has been perforated with tumour spreading into adjacent soft tissues (Figs. 2.14, *page 17*, 2.15, *page 18*).

If teeth are present their relationship with the lesion should be recorded as well as whether root resorption has occurred. In the case of gingival tumours one should determine whether the lesion arises from the buccal or the palatal surface of the gingiva (Fig. 2.16, *page 20*).

Specific Features

If the specimen contains teeth it will be helpful to use the two-digit numerical notation for teeth as used in dentistry for recording numbers and types of teeth that are present. In this notation the first digit indicates the part of the jaw and the second the place in the teeth row (Fig. 2.17, *page 21*). Moreover, this method of notation facilitates identification of sites from which samples for histological investigation are taken.

Buccal gingival cancers may cross the vestibular fold and involve the mucosal lining of the adjacent cheek. Another possibility is submucosal lateral spread into the adjacent cheek musculature (Figs. 2.18, 2.19, *page 22*). Squamous cell cancer of the anterior gingiva may cross the anterior vestibular fold and extend into the mucosal lining of the inner surface of the upper lip or may spread submucosally into the lip musculature (Figs. 2.20–2.23, *page 23–25*).

If squamous cell cancer involves the maxillary tuberosity, there may be submucosal tumour spread dorsally into the pterygoid musculature and infratemporal fossa. Extending the frontal slices dorsally beyond the mucosa-covered palatal surface of the specimen allows analysis of this part of the maxillary specimen. These dorsal slices will also allow examination of the pterygopalatine fossa for the presence of tumour spread in this area (Fig. 2.24, *page 26*).

Macroscopic appearance of intraosseous maxillary tumours.

a Cut surface of hemimaxillectomy to treat osteosarcoma. The tumour can be seen bulging into the maxillary sinus.

b Hemimaxillectomy with osteosarcoma that penetrates into the buccal as well as palatal soft tissues.

c Haematoxylin and eosin stained mounted section of the specimen shown in **b.** Soft tissue extension is clearly visible.

d Buccopalatal slices from a partial maxillectomy to treat ossifying fibroma.

e Haematoxylin and eosin stained mounted section to illustrate the circumscribed character of the lesion shown in **d.**

Figure 2.15
◄

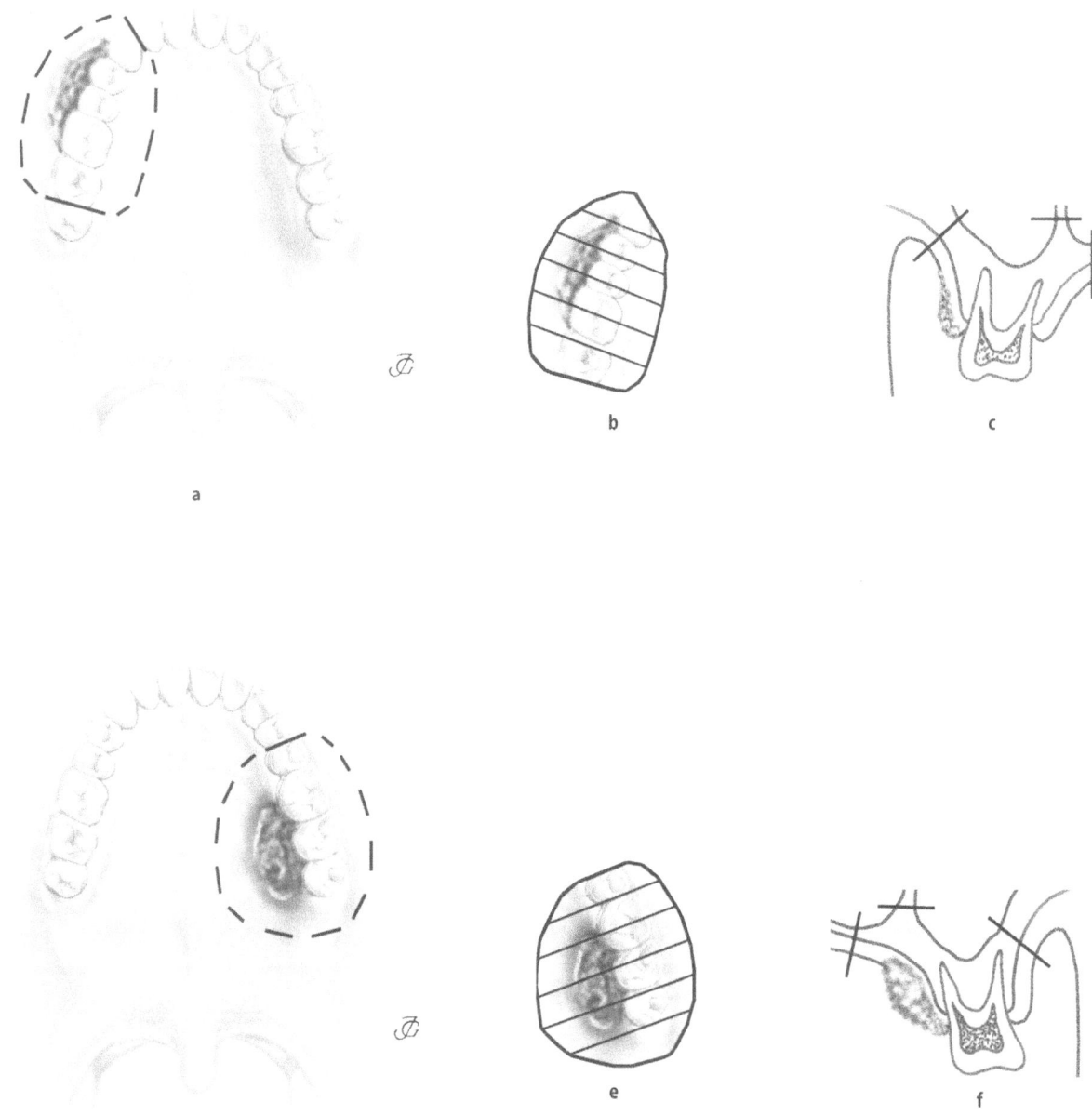

Figure 2.16
▲

Pathological anatomy of gingival cancer located either buccally or palatally.

a Clinical appearance of buccal gingival cancer and outline of the resection.

b Surgical specimen of buccal gingival cancer with plane of sectioning.

c Cut surface and outline of the resection of the specimen with buccal gingival cancer.

d Clinical appearance of palatal gingival cancer and outline of the resection.

e Surgical specimen of palatal gingival cancer with plane of sectioning.

f Cut surface and outline of the resection of the specimen with palatal gingival cancer.

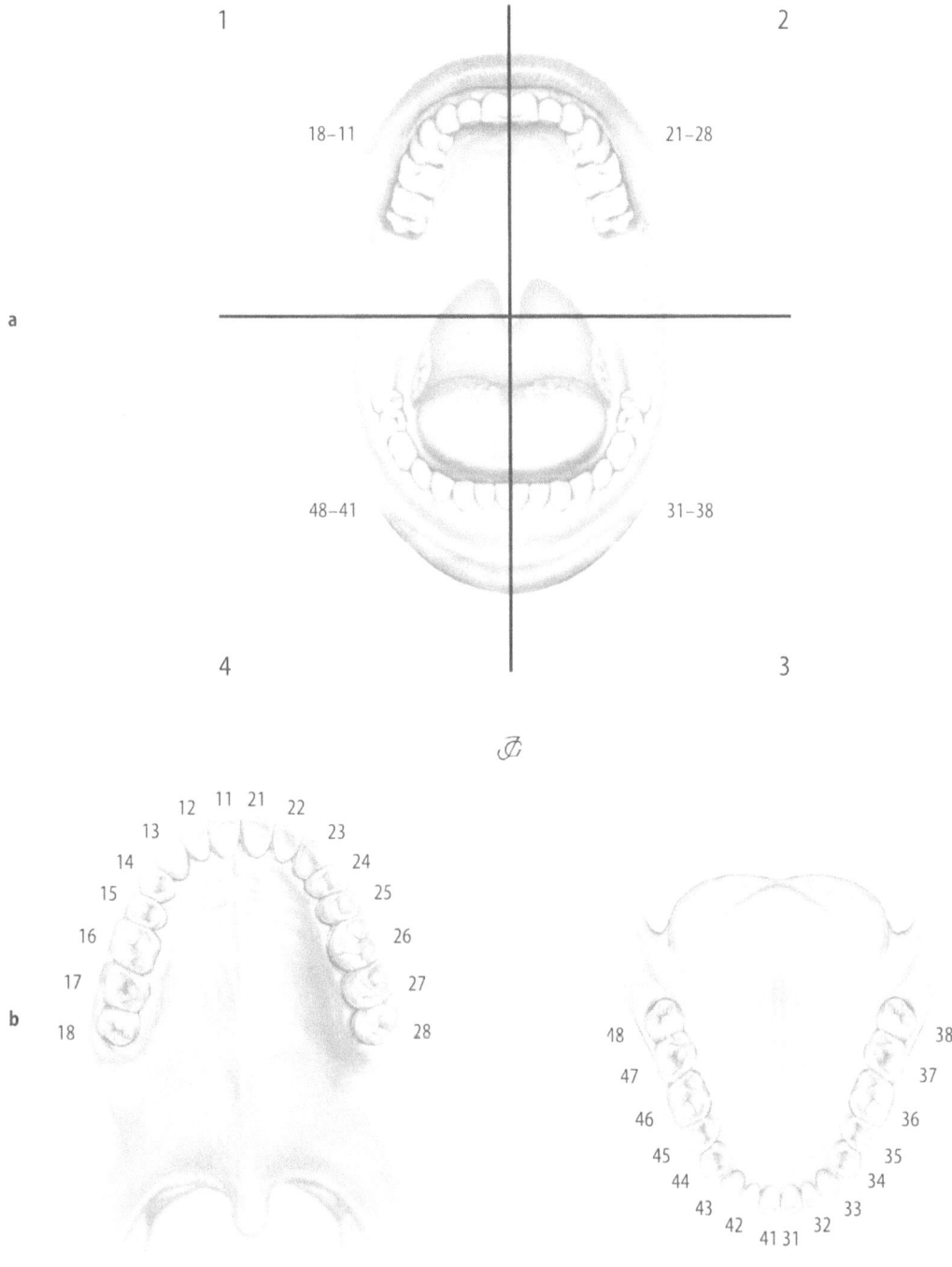

Diagrams to illustrate the two-digit teeth notation that may be used by clinicians to indicate sites from which lesions submitted for examination are taken and that can be employed by the pathologist in identifying the site of samples taken for microscopy.

a System depicted according to jaw quadrant, upper right teeth lying in quadrant 1, upper left teeth in quadrant 2, lower left teeth in quadrant 3 and lower right teeth in quadrant 4.

b Notation for each individual tooth. The first digit refers to quadrant; the second digit refers to place in the teeth row.

Figure 2.17
▲

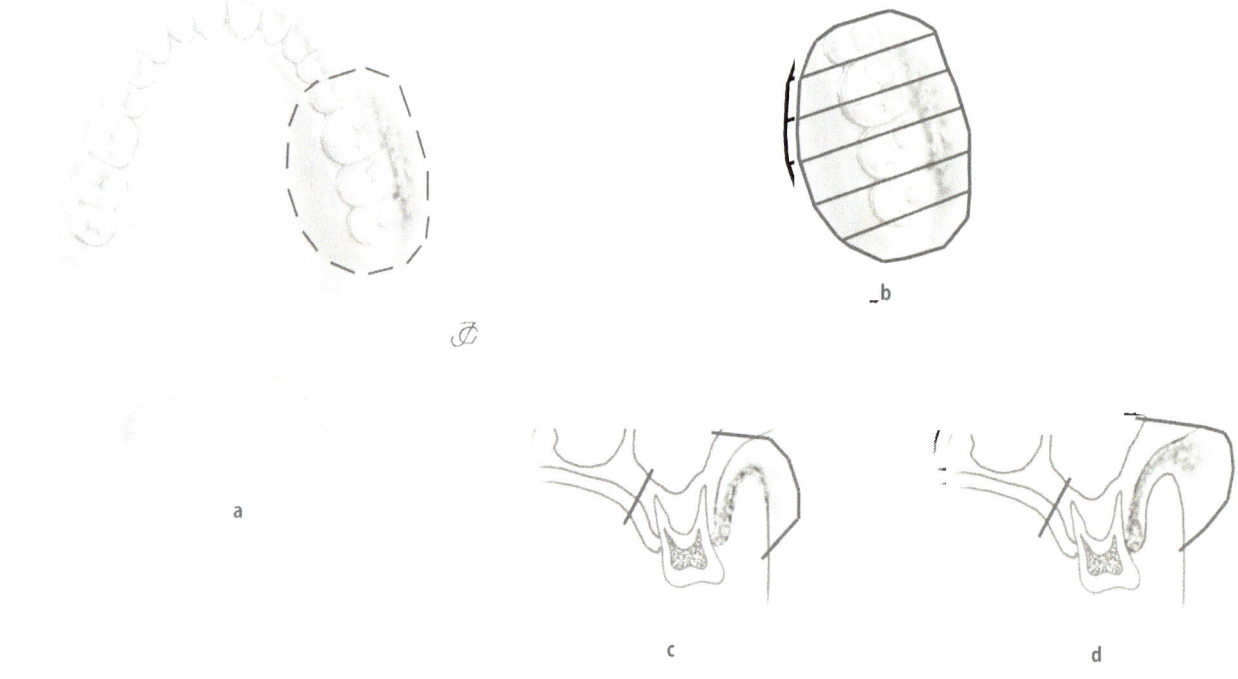

Figure 2.18
▲

Pathological anatomy of buccal gingival cancer spreading into the cheek.

a Clinical appearance and outline of the resection.

b Surgical specimen and plane of sectioning.

c Frontal view showing intramucosal spread into the cheek.

d Frontal view showing submucosal spread into the cheek musculature.

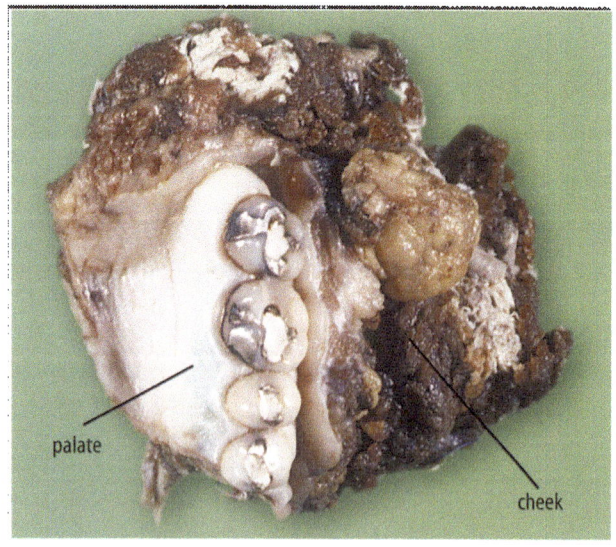

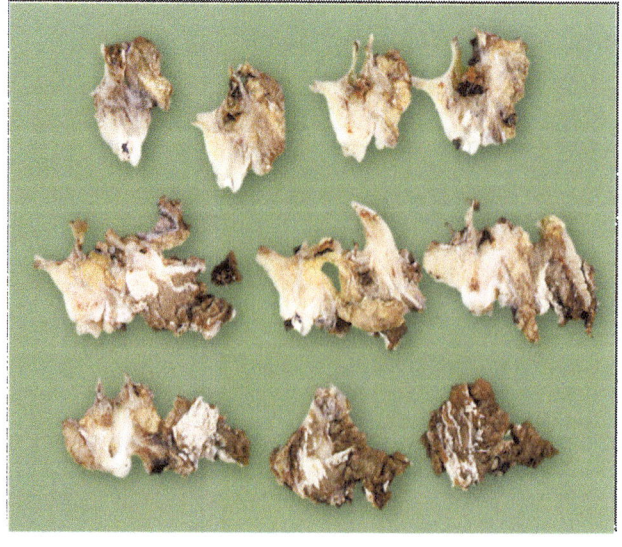

a

b

Figure 2.19

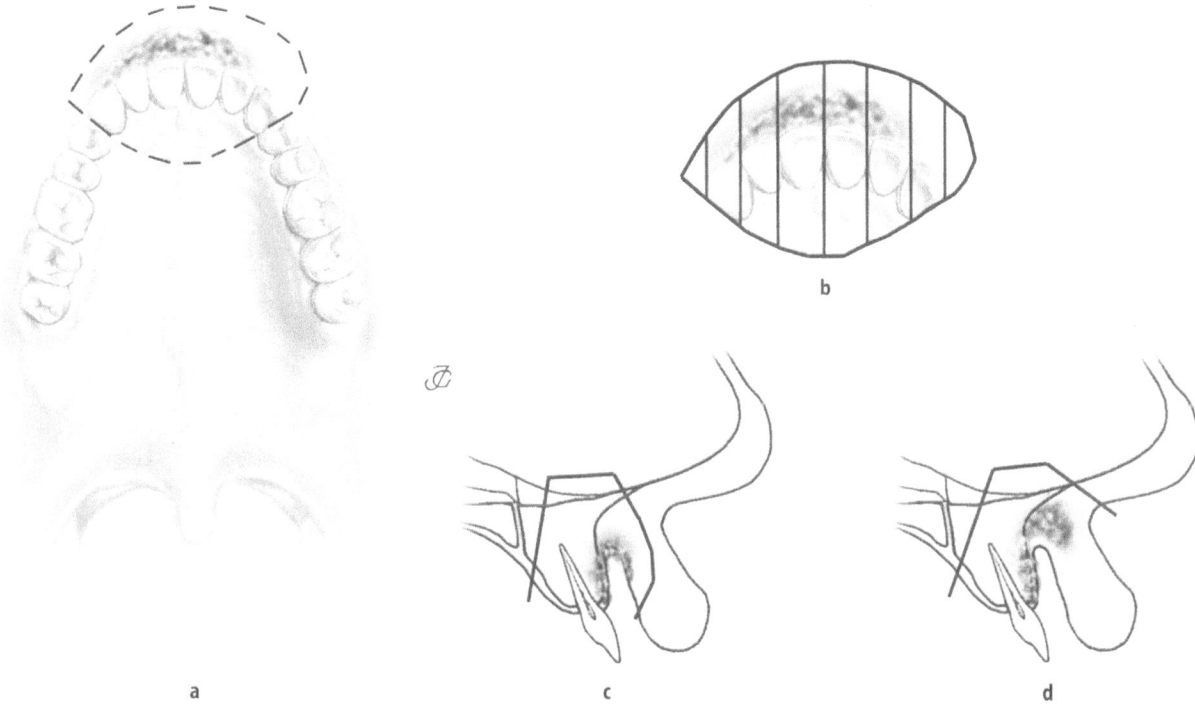

a

b

c

d

Pathological anatomy of labial gingival cancer spreading into the upper lip.

a Clinical appearance and outline of the resection.

b Surgical specimen and plane of sectioning.

c Cut surface showing intramucosal spread into the lip mucosa and outline of the resection.

d Cut surface showing submucosal spread into the lip musculature and outline of the resection. In this case the specimen includes the upper lip.

Figure 2.20
▲

Macroscopic appearance of buccal gingival cancer extending into the cheek.

a Palatal view of specimen.

b Slices cut buccopalatally to display tumour extension laterally into the soft tissues of the cheek.

Figure 2.19
◄

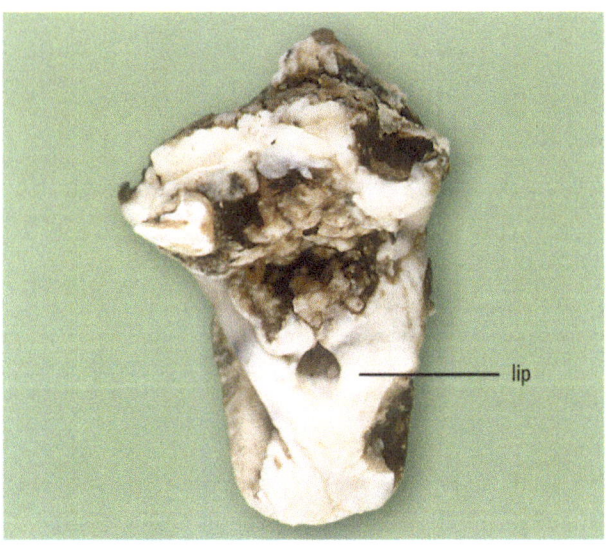

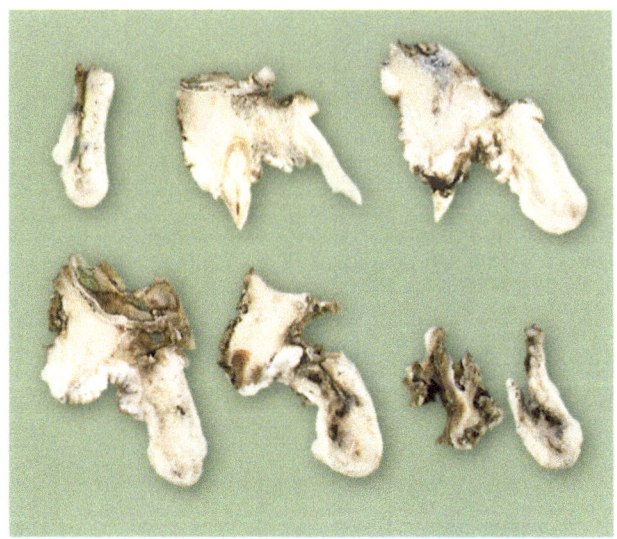

lip

a

b

Figure 2.21 ▲ Macroscopic appearance of cancer at the anterior alveolar maxillary process spreading into the upper lip.

a Posterior view of specimen showing tumour spreading from the partly edentulous anterior maxillary alveolar process into the inner side of the upper lip.

b Same specimen cut ventrodorsally to display tumour site and extension.

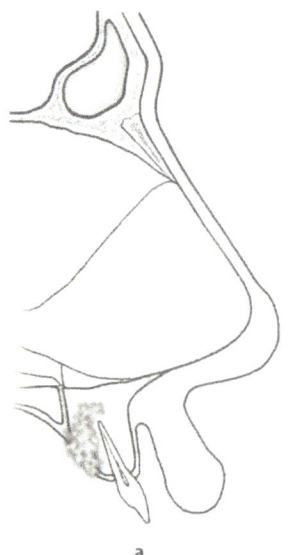

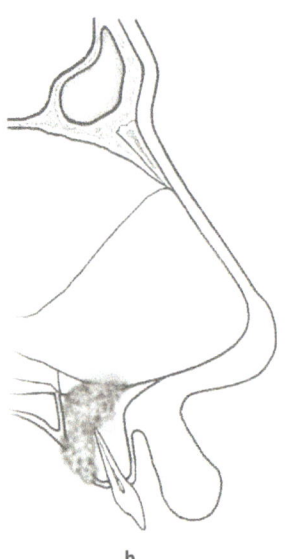

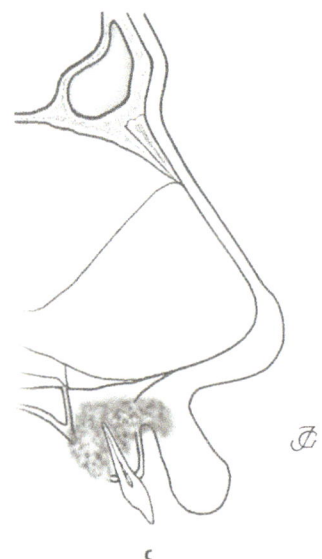

a

b

c

Figure 2.22

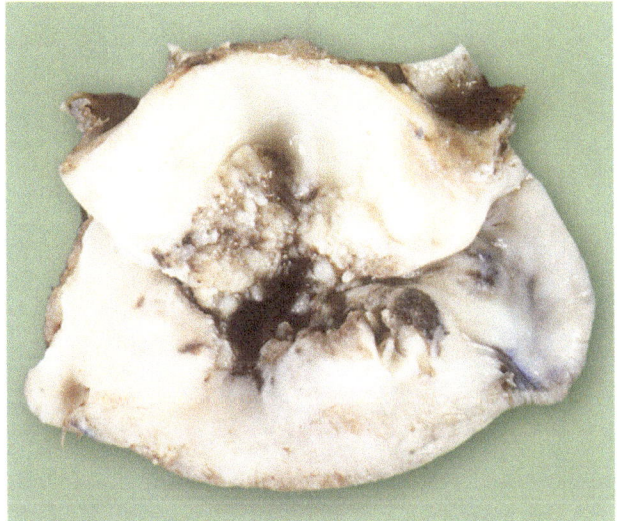

a

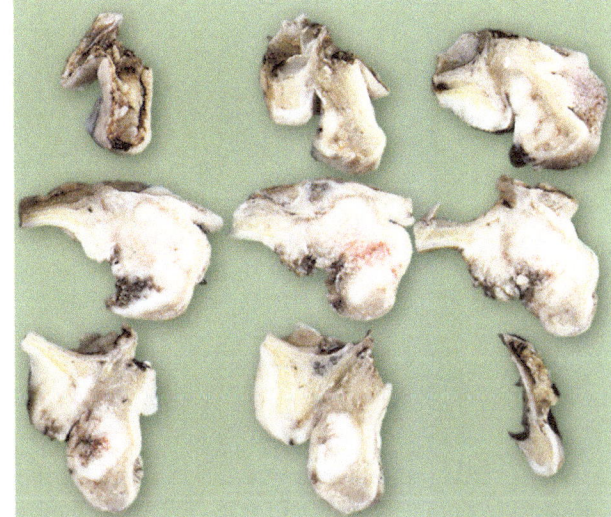

b

Macroscopic appearance of anterior alveolar process cancer extending into the upper lip.

a Palatal view showing ulcerating tumour at the edentulous anterior alveolar process of the maxilla and the adjacent side of the upper lip.

b Slices cut ventrodorsally showing extensive tumour spread in the upper lip.

Figure 2.23
▲

Sagittal drawings to illustrate different routes that may be taken by cancer of the anterior maxilla.

a Tumour confined to the mucosa and underlying bone.

b Tumour penetrating through the floor of the nose into the nasal cavity.

c Tumour growing ventrally through the bone into the musculature of the upper lip.

Figure 2.22
◄

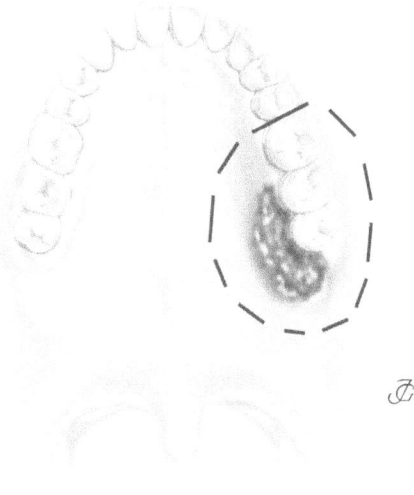

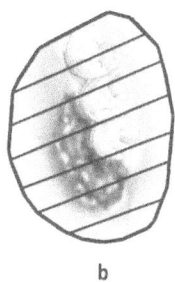

b

a

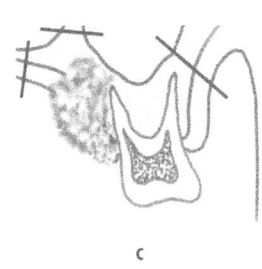

c

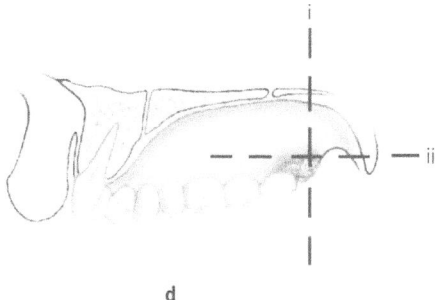

d

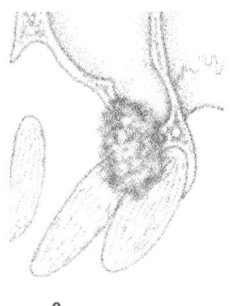

e

Figure 2.24
▲

Pathological anatomy of cancer at the maxillary tuberosity spreading dorsally into the pterygoid area.

a Clinical appearance and outline of the resection.

b Surgical specimen and plane of sectioning.

c Cut surface and outline of the resection.

d Median sagittal view. In projection plane i the cut surface is as shown in **c**; in projection plane ii the cut surface is as shown in **e**, which displays the dorsal spread into pterygoid bone and muscle.

Mandible

Anatomy

The mandible consists of a horseshoe-shaped bone. It can be divided into one horizontal part, the body with superimposed alveolar ridge that is the tooth-bearing part, and two vertical parts, the ascending rami. In the oral cavity it is covered by the mucosa of the vestibular fold laterally and anteriorly and the mucosa of the floor of the mouth medially. Between the two mucosal surfaces lies the strip of alveolar ridge mucosa that, as for the maxilla, is tightly connected with the underlying mandibular bone and that surrounds the necks of the mandibular teeth. The dorsal border of the alveolar ridge mucosa lies at the junction with the retromolar trigone. At the inner surface of the ascending ramus, at the mandibular foramen, the lower alveolar nerve enters the mandibular body where this nerve lies in the mandibular canal. At the mental foramen the nerve leaves the mandible to become the sensory nerve of the lower lip.

Specimen

Resections containing mandibular bone are usually done for squamous cell cancers arising in the gingiva or in adjacent mucosal linings so close to the mandible that bone resection is needed to ensure an adequate margin. Rarer lesions necessitating mandibular resection are the same neoplasms as occur in the maxilla, salivary gland tumours excepted. Mandibular resections may vary in size. They can grossly be divided into two main groups: those in which the continuity of the mandible is sacrificed and those in which parts of the mandible are removed while saving the lower border and thus maintaining the integrity of the bone. Within this simplified scheme, many modifications are possible (Fig. 2.25, page 28). In the case of the so-called through and through resection, two bone margins, both vertical, have to be assessed, whereas in the case of mandibular resections that save the lower border by only removing parts of the mandibular body and the alveolar ridge, one has also to investigate the horizontal bone margin. Tumours may spread alongside the lower alveolar nerve. In the case of complete resection of the mandibular body one should identify the cut surface of the nerve in the posterior bone margin for histological examination to assess whether this margin is tumour-free. Sometimes the dorsal osteotomy line lies dorsal to the mandibular foramen. In that case the nerve should be identified at its entrance site in the mandibular bone and subsequently dissected cranially to sample its extraosseous cut surface for histology. When the lower mandibular border is saved one should assess whether the nerve is contained within the removed specimen, in which case the rules as mentioned above apply. When the nerve lies below the horizontal osteotomy margin it is left in situ, and thus does not form part of the specimen.

Dissection

Examination of the mandibular specimen starts with recording externally visible features. In the case of a mucosal lesion one should determine location and size. In the case of intraosseous lesions one should see whether there is any externally visible bony swelling and if the swelling is due to cortical expansion. Finally, one should assess the type of mandibular resection that has been done.

The best way to dissect a mandibular specimen is to cut slices perpendicular to the long axis of the mandibular body using the water-cooled diamond saw. In the posterior part of the jaw this means slicing parallel to the frontal plane (Figs. 2.26, page 29, 2.27, page 30); in the anterior part of the jaw this means slicing parallel to the sagittal plane (Figs. 2.28, page 30, 2.29, page 31). In the case of specimens containing the cuspid–premolar region one has to follow the curve of the alveolar ridge. This means that in this area, slices have to be made that in turn are wedge-shaped displaying the surgical margin facing the oral vestibule and are full-thickness showing the lingual surgical margin as well (Fig. 2.30, page 32).

Slices thus obtained exhibit a full view of the entire thickness of mandibular bone and covering mucosa. They allow assessment of the way in which lesions in covering alveolar ridge mucosa involve underlying bone, as well as measurement of their thickness and depth of penetration. In the case of intraosseous lesions one should use these slices to measure the size of the lesion and to record whether the lesion has caused expansion and/or attenuation of adjacent cortical bone or whether the tumour a

b

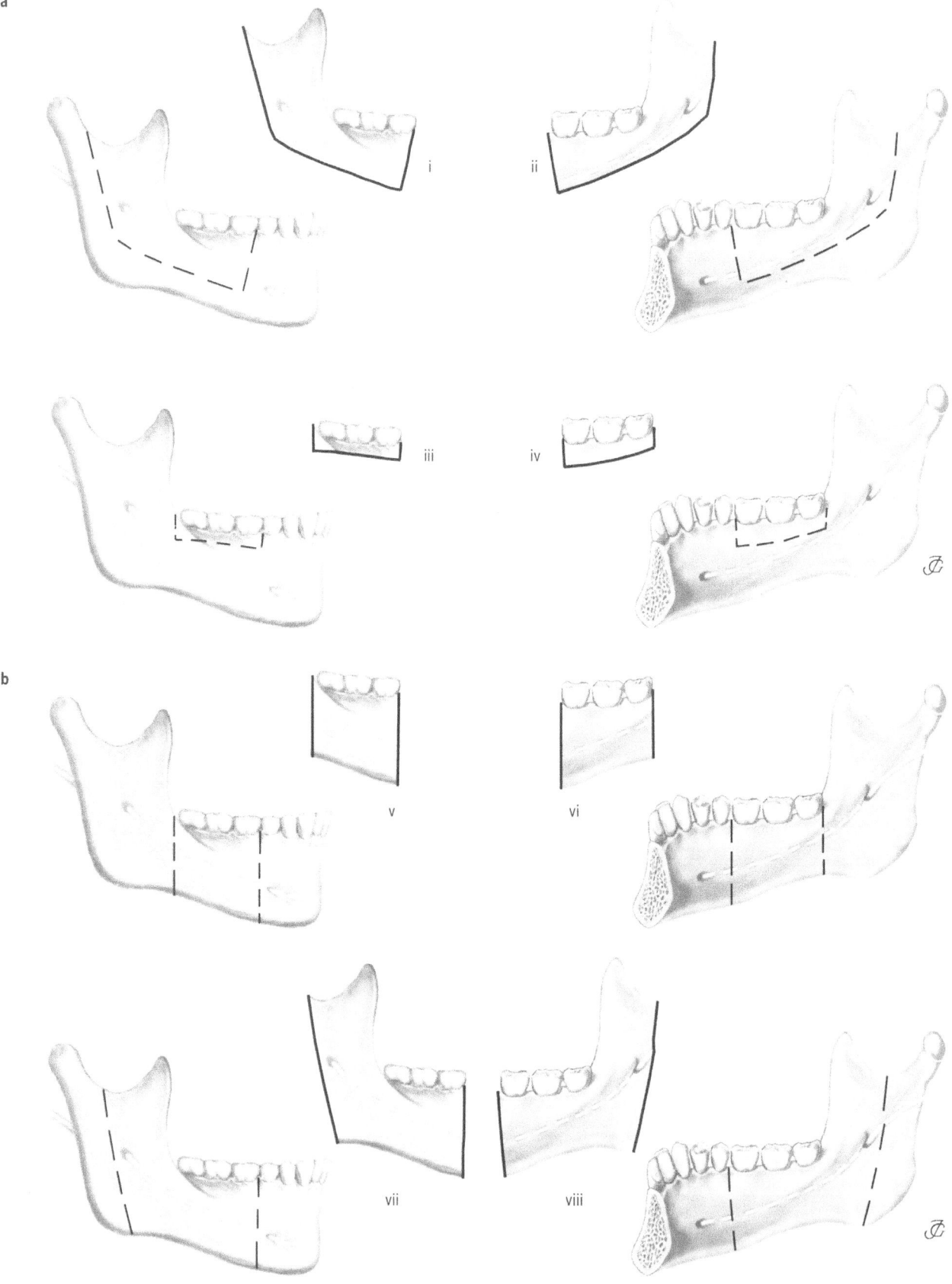

Figure 2.25

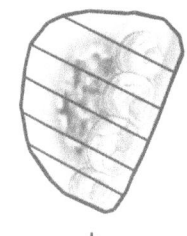

b

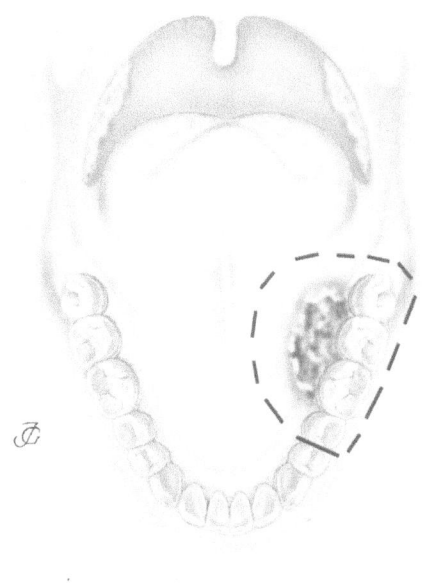

a

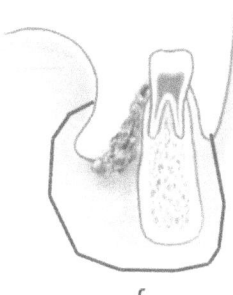

c

Pathological anatomy of lingual gingival cancer in the posterior area of the mandible.

a Clinical appearance and outline of the resection.

b Surgical specimen and plane of sectioning.

c Cut surface exhibiting tumour thickness and relationship with surrounding structures as well as the outline of the resection. The specimen includes the entire height of the mandible.

Figure 2.26
▲

Schematic drawing displaying various types of mandibular osteotomies in relation to the lower alveolar nerve.

a Types of osteotomies that maintain the continuity of the mandible.

b Types of osteotomies in which the continuity of the mandible is sacrificed. When saving the lower mandibular border, the so-called segmental osteotomy, the resected part may include the lower alveolar nerve (i, ii) or may consist of the alveolar process only, leaving the nerve in situ (iii, iv). In the case of through and through osteotomies, the posterior osteotomy line may lie anterior (v, vi) or posterior (vii, viii) to the mandibular foramen. These figures show in which instances the alveolar nerve lies in the osteotomy line and thus has to be examined for peri-neural tumour spread. In **a** and **b** the left vertical row displays the lateral surface of the mandible, the right vertical row displays the medial surface.

Figure 2.25
◄

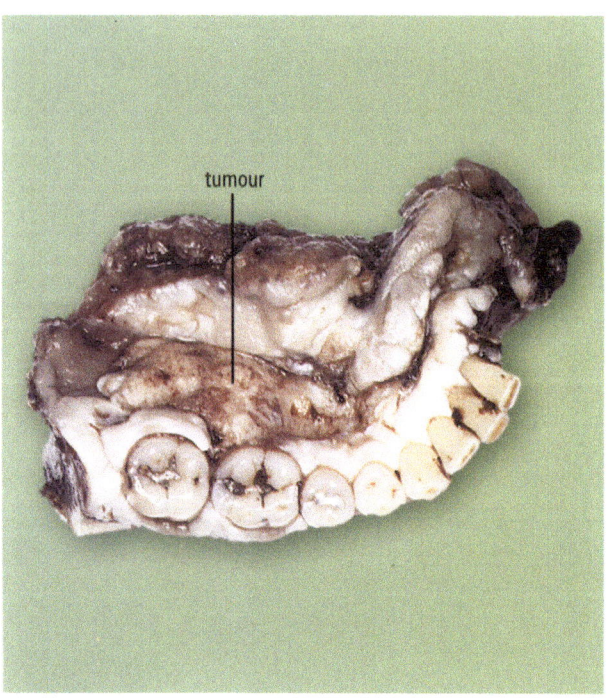

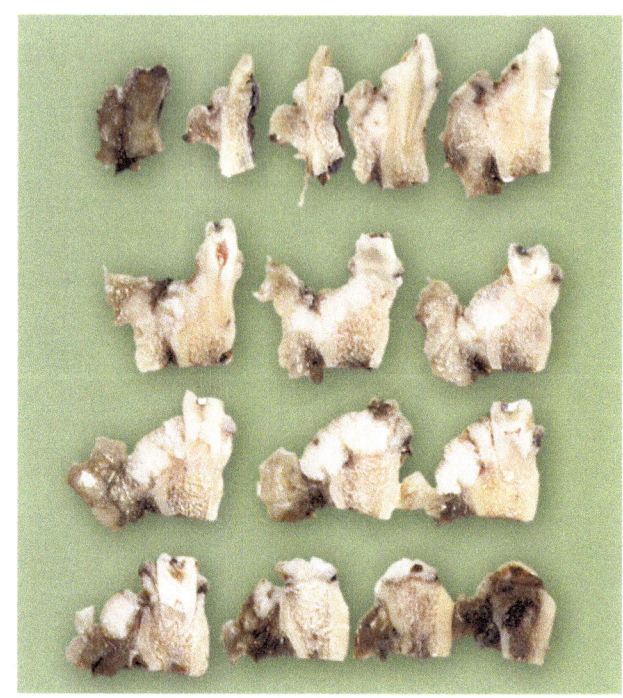

a

b

Figure 2.27 ▲ Macroscopic appearance of lingually located gingival cancer in the mandible.

a Occlusal view showing tumour at the lingual side of the molar teeth extending into the adjacent floor of the mouth.

b Slices obtained when cutting the specimen buccolingually. Tumour can be seen destroying the lingual part of the tooth-bearing part of the mandibular alveolar process. In this case tumour extension allowed a restricted mandibulectomy. Therefore the specimen contains only the cranial half of the mandible, the lower part with its cortical border being left in situ.

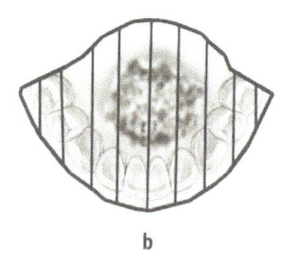

b

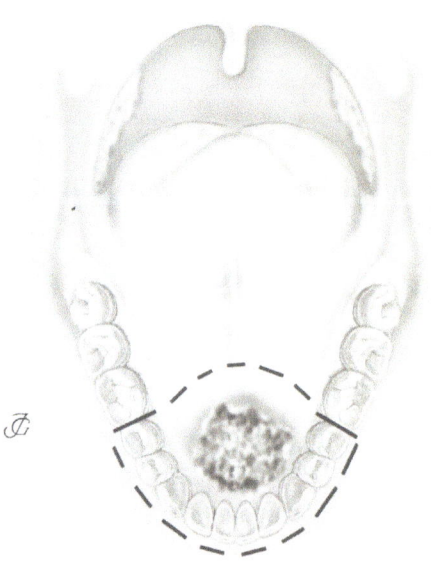

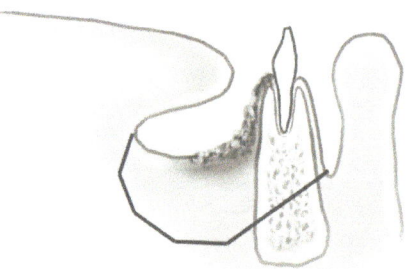

a

c

Figure 2.28

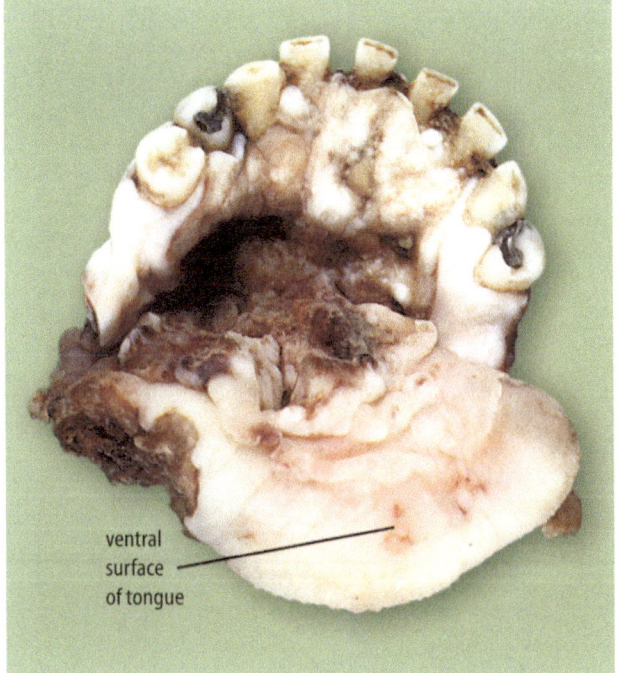

ventral
surface
of tongue

a

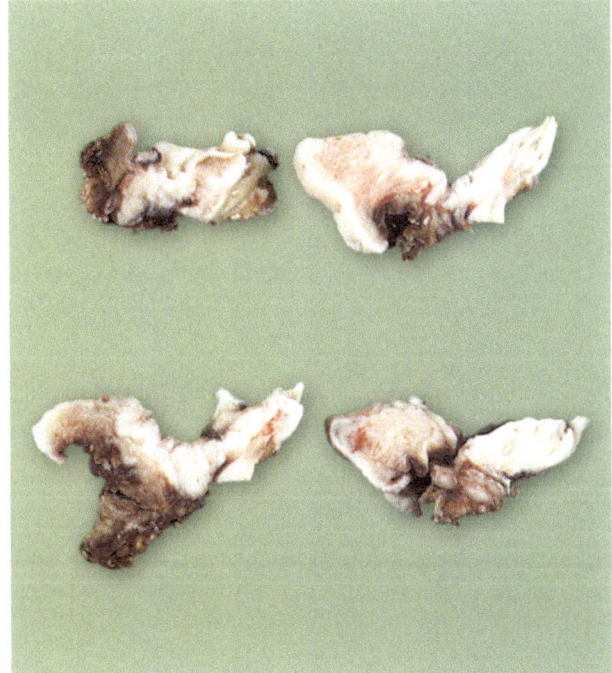

b

Macroscopic appearance of anterior lingual gingival cancer spreading into the adjacent anterior part of the mouth.

a Posterior view showing ulcerating tumour mass occupying the lingual gingival border as well as the floor of the mouth. The ventral surface of the tongue is reflected to allow visualisation of the tumour.

b Slices made ventrodorsally displaying tumour site and extension.

Figure 2.29
▲

Pathological anatomy of lingual gingival cancer in the anterior area of the mandible.

a Clinical appearance and outline of the resection.

b Surgical specimen and plane of sectioning.

c Cut surface exhibiting tumour thickness and relationship with surrounding structures as well as the outline of the resection. In this case the lower part of the mandibular bone is left in situ.

Figure 2.28
◄

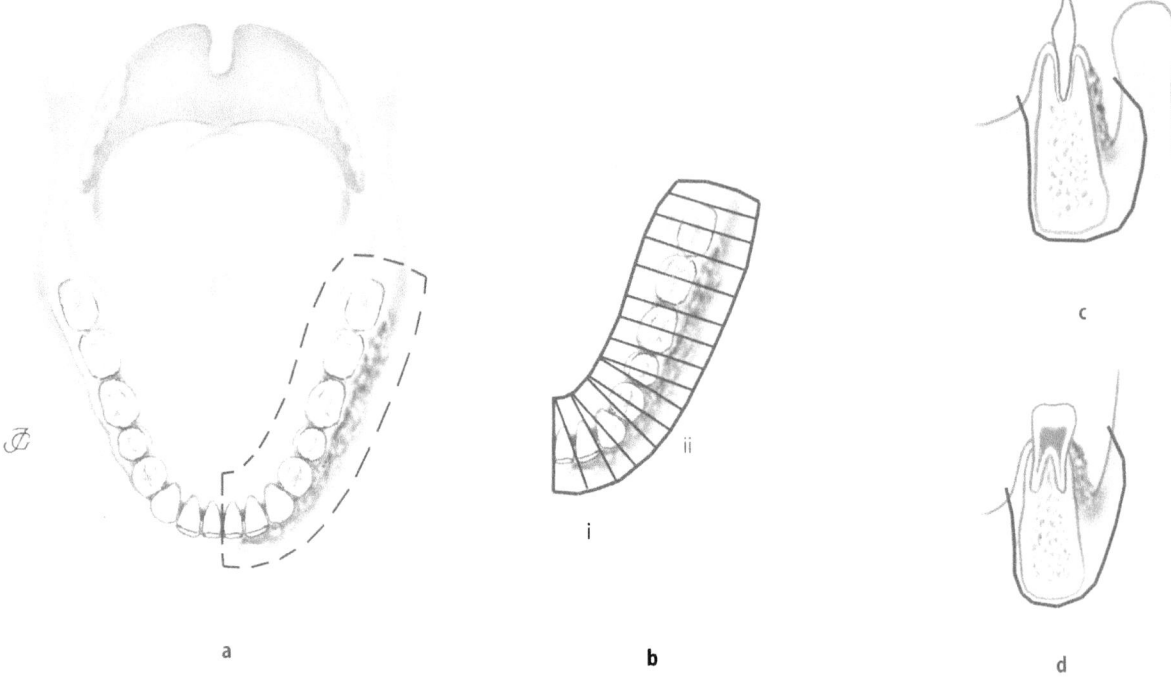

a

b

c

d

Figure 2.30
▲

Pathological anatomy of buccal gingival cancer in the mandible that involves the anterior as well as the posterior part.

a Clinical appearance and outline of the resection.

b Surgical specimen with plane of sectioning that rotates to accommodate the parabolic teeth row. In the cuspid–premolar area slices are alternating full-thickness (i) and wedge-shaped (ii).

c Cut surface and outline of the resection anteriorly.

d Cut surface and outline of the resection posteriorly.

Figure 2.32
▶

Macroscopic appearances of intraosseous mandibular tumour.

a Cut surface showing chondrosarcoma penetrating from the medullary cavity through the buccal cortex into adjacent soft tissues.

b Mounted haematoxylin and eosin stained section from the same specimen as in **a** showing tumour extension. The tumour has also caused partial resorption of the involved tooth.

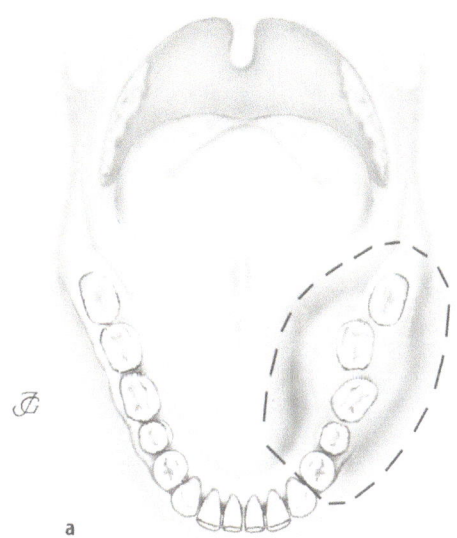

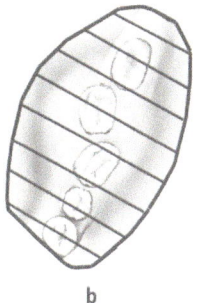

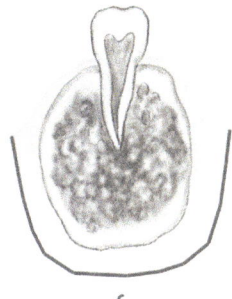

Pathological anatomy of intraosseous mandibular tumour.

a Clinical appearance and outline of the resection.

b Surgical specimen and plane of sectioning.

c Cut surface that shows the relationship between tumour and surrounding structures as well as the outline of the resection. Osseous and odontogenic tumours may show this pattern.

Figure 2.31
▲

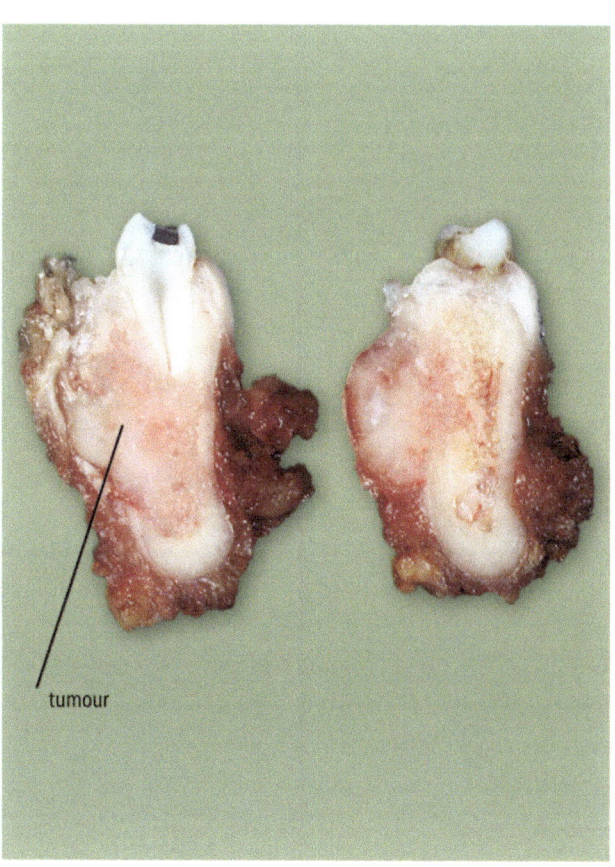

a

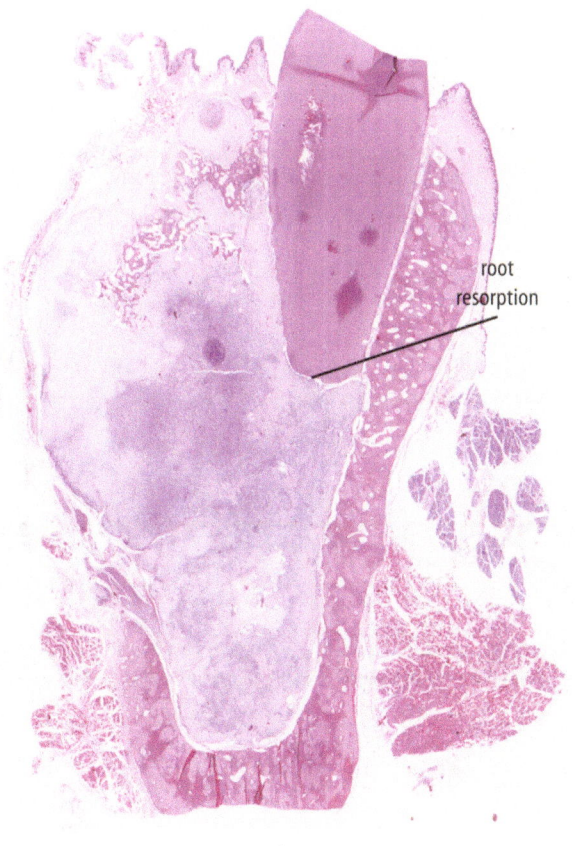

root resorption

b

Figure 2.32

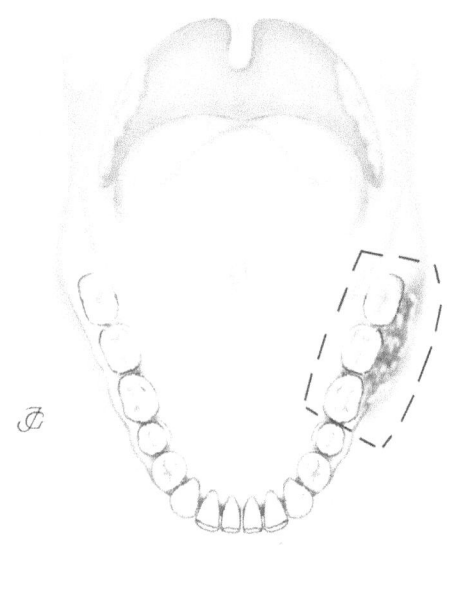

a

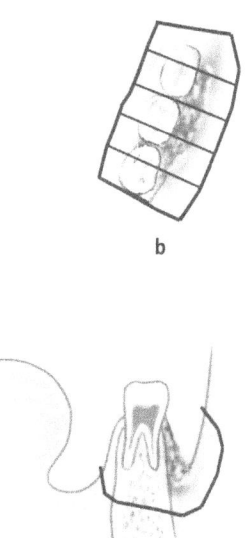

b

c

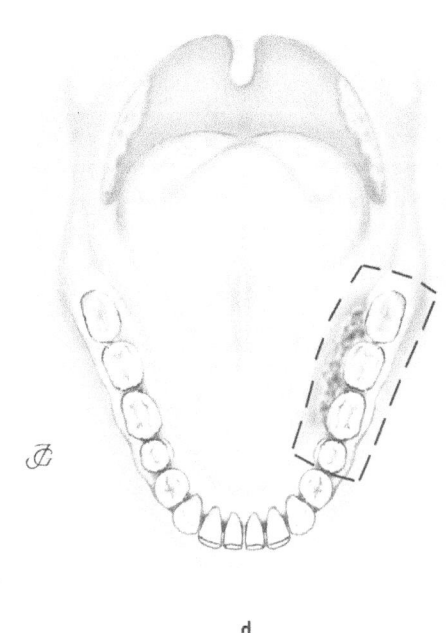

d

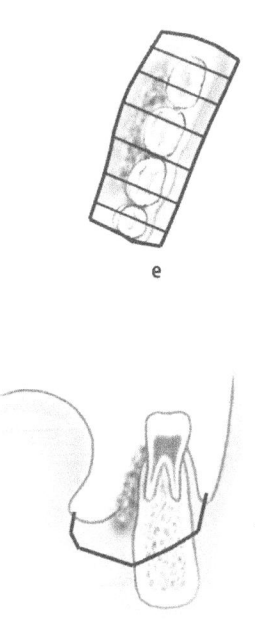

e

f

Figure 2.33

perforates through the cortical bone either lingually or buccally. One should also record whether there is any relationship between an intraosseous lesion and roots of teeth present in the resected specimen; this is especially important when dealing with fibroosseous or odontogenic lesions. Just as for the maxillary teeth, one should look for the presence of root resorption (Figs. 2.31, 2.32, page 33).

Specific Features

In the case of squamous cell cancer of the mandibular gingiva one should record whether the tumour is buccally or lingually located (Fig. 2.33). Moreover, one should assess the relationship between tumour and underlying mandibular bone and, if present, teeth. As for the maxilla, the two-digit dental tooth notation may be useful in this respect.

The way the tumour involves bone may vary considerably. Bone may be resorbed over a broad front or the tumour may penetrate diffusely into the bone marrow. Bone destruction may be in either a horizontal or a vertical direction and there may also be diffuse periosteal involvement (Figs. 2.34, page 36, 2.35, page 37). Surgeons pay much attention to the preoperative assessment of bone involvement by tumour to know whether bone-saving surgery is feasible, and it is the responsibility of the pathologist to dissect the specimen in such a way that the preoperative findings concerning bone involvement can be evaluated. Especially when bone is destroyed laterally, radiographs will underscore the extent of bone destruction.

In the case of intraosseous mandibular tumours it may be useful to split the specimen along its long axis after having taken anterior and posterior frontal slices to investigate the bony resection margins. This way of cutting the specimen allows comparison of macroscopic tumour spread with the data provided by panoramic radiographs, the so-called orthopantomogram (Figs. 2.36, page 38, 2.37, page 39).

Quite often, lingually located squamous cell cancer spreads into the adjacent floor of the mouth. In these instances the combined rules for dissecting mandibular as well as floor of mouth specimens apply (Figs. 2.38, page 39, 2.39, page 40). Similar to buccally located gingival cancer in the upper jaw, there may be crossing of the oral vestibule and involvement of the mucosal lining of the cheek or inner surface of the lip, in this instance the lower lip (Figs. 2.40, page 40, 2.41, page 41).

Retromolar Trigone

Anatomy

The retromolar trigone or retromolar area consists of a triangular mucosal surface that lines the ventral surface of the ascending mandibular ramus. Ventrocaudally it is bordered by the gingiva posterior to the last molar tooth in the mandible, mostly the third, and ventrocranially by the mucosa covering the maxillary tuberosity. Its lateral and medial borders are respectively the buccal mucosa and the anterior faucial pillar.

Specimen

Resections of the retromolar area are usually done for treatment of squamous cell cancer in this area.

Pathological anatomy of gingival cancers in the posterior mandible.

a Clinical appearance and outline of the resection of buccal gingival cancer.

b Surgical specimen and plane of sectioning.

c Cut surface and outline of the resection.

d Clinical appearance and outline of the resection of lingual gingival cancer.

e Surgical specimen and plane of sectioning.

f Cut surface and outline of the resection. The tumour dimensions determine whether it is possible to save parts of the mandibular bone as shown in **c** and **f**.

Figure 2.33
◄

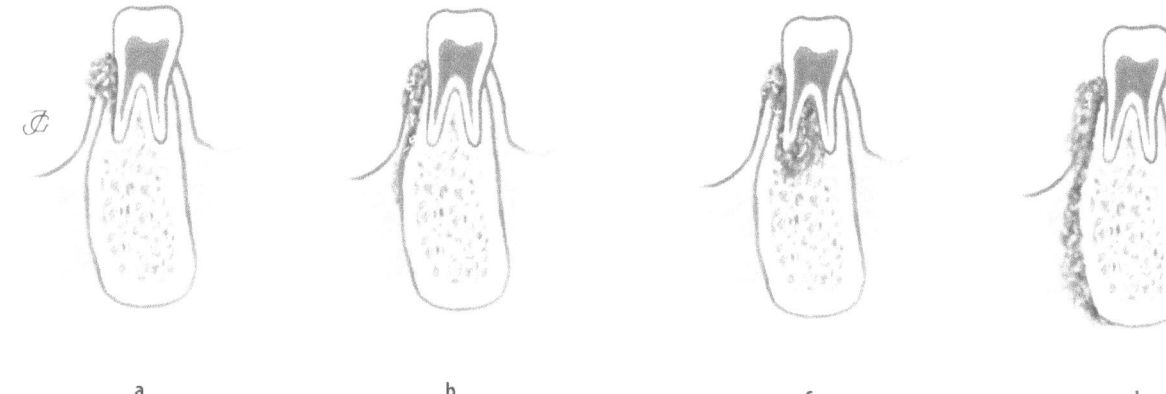

a   b   c   d

Figure 2.34   Patterns of mandibular bone involvement by gingival cancer.
▲
a Tumour resorbs bone in a vertical direction, thus reducing the height of the dental socket.

b Tumour erodes bone horizontally, thus reducing the thickness of the alveolar socket wall without reducing its height.

c Tumour spreads through the alveolar ligament space.

d Tumour grows downward into the mandibular periosteum without bone resorption. Only in situation **a** will radiographs reflect the real extent of bone involvement by tumour. In all other instances the extent of bone involvement by tumour will be underestimated when relying on the radiographs.

Figure 2.35   Macroscopic appearance of bone destruction by cancer adjacent to the mandible.
▶
a Tumour surrounding the teeth and destroying the upper part of the alveolar process.

b Tumour lateral to the cranial part of the alveolar socket and causing superficial bone erosion.

c Tumour involving the periodontal ligament space.

d Tumour spreading into the lingual periosteum without causing bone destruction.

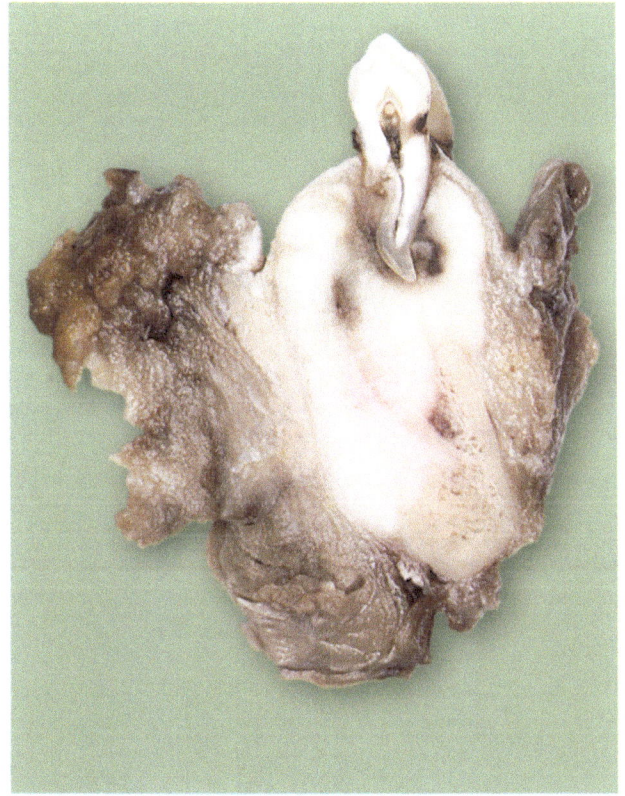

a

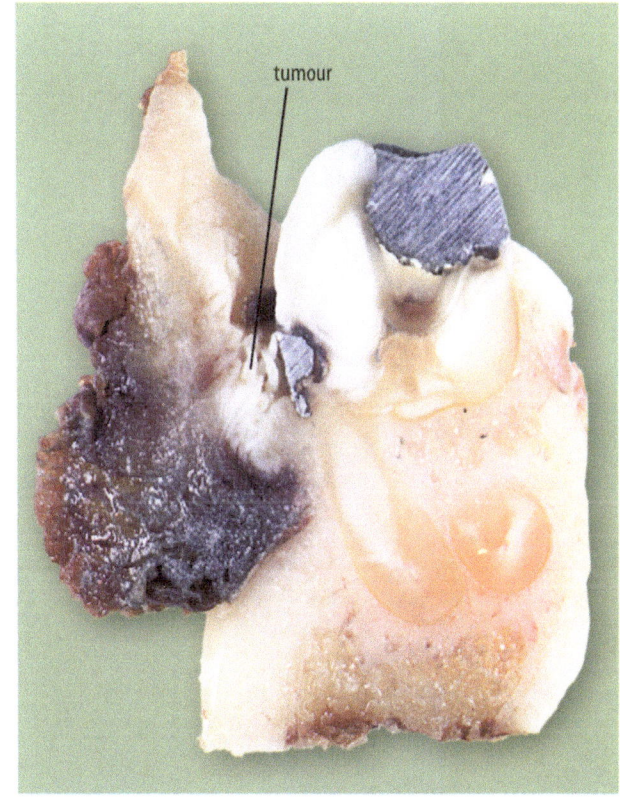

b

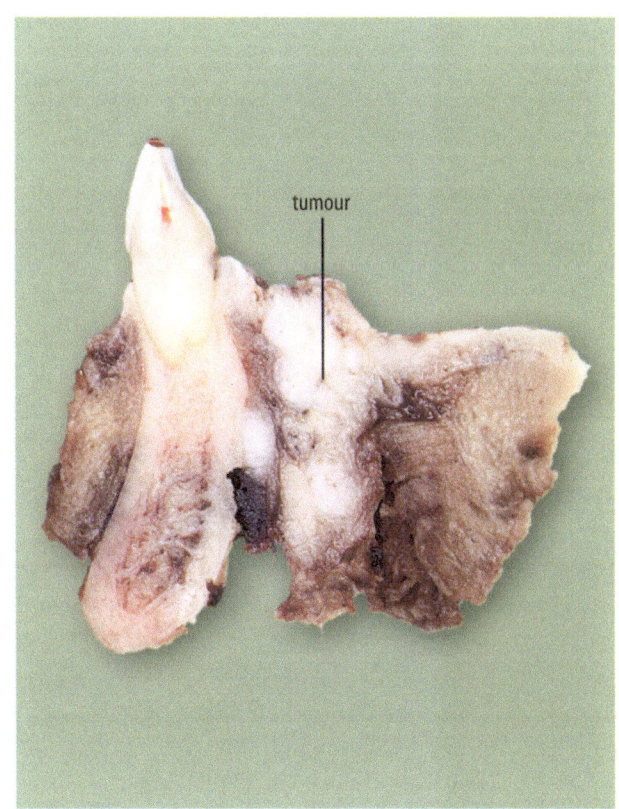

c

d

Figure 2.35

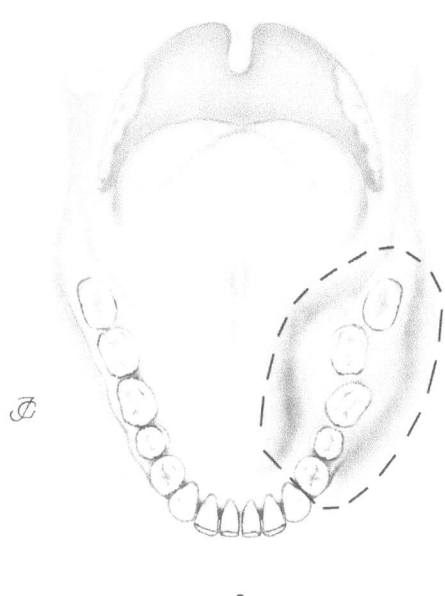

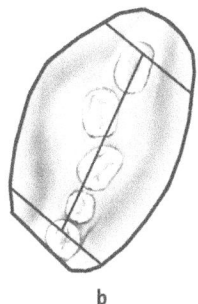

b

a

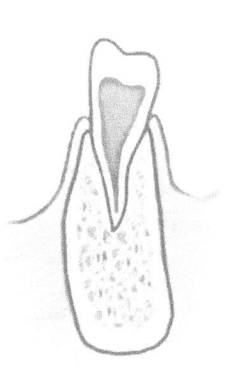

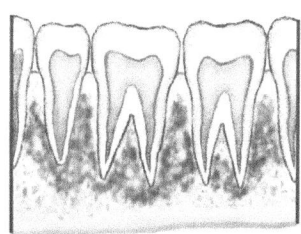

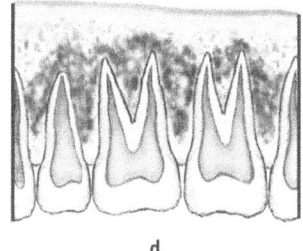

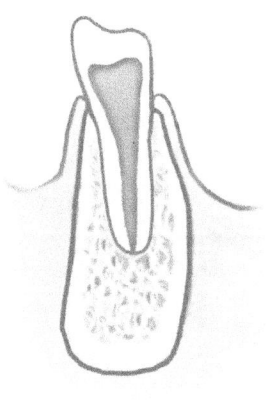

c

d

e

Figure 2.36
▲

Pathological anatomy of intraosseous mandibular tumour.

a Clinical appearance and outline of the resection.

b Surgical specimen and plane of sectioning. Note that after making full-thickness slices from the anterior and posterior border, the intermediate part of the specimen is split into a lingual half and a buccal half along its median axis.

c Cut surface of an anterior slice.

d Cut surfaces of intermediate part.

e Cut surface of a posterior slice. This method allows correlation of macroscopic tumour extension with panoramic radiographs obtained preoperatively.

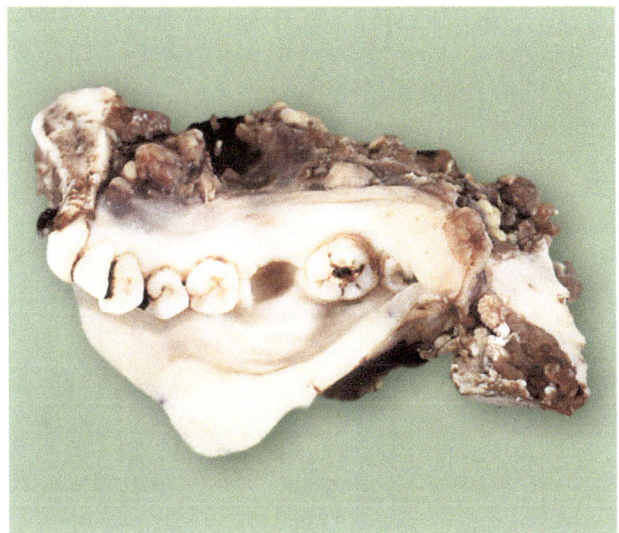

a

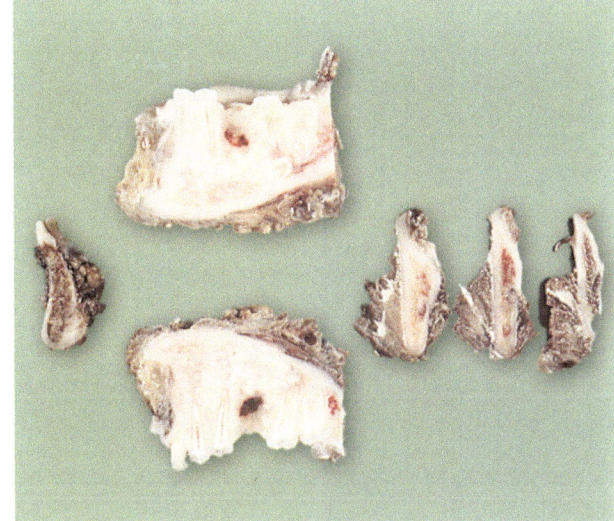

b

Macroscopic appearance of mandibular osteosarcoma, handled as shown in Fig. 2.36.

a Occlusal view of specimen. Tumour can be seen bulging buccally.

b Specimen dissected by cutting slices buccolingually ventrally and dorsally, and by splitting the intermediate part into a buccal and a lingual half.

Figure 2.37
▲

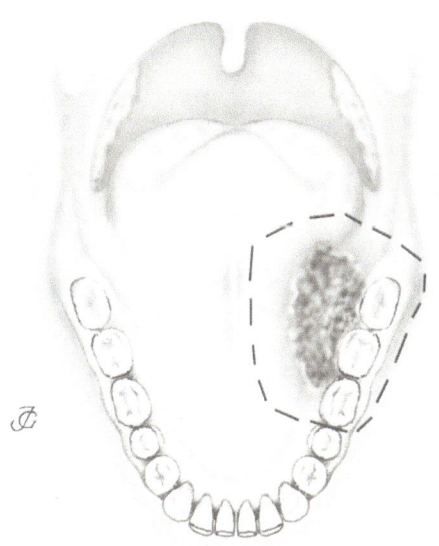

a

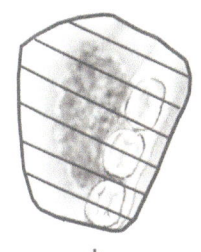

b

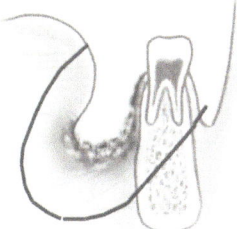

c

Pathological anatomy of lingual gingival cancer spreading into the adjacent floor of the mouth.

a Clinical appearance and outline of the resection.

b Surgical specimen and plane of sectioning.

c Cut surface showing tumour thickness and involvement of adjacent structures.

Figure 2.38
▲

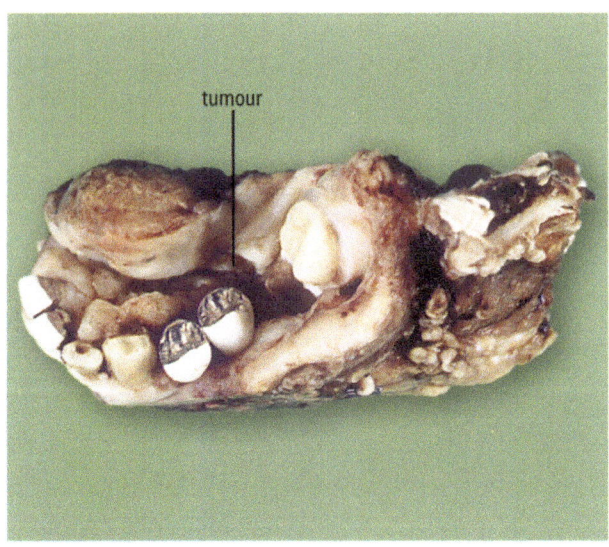

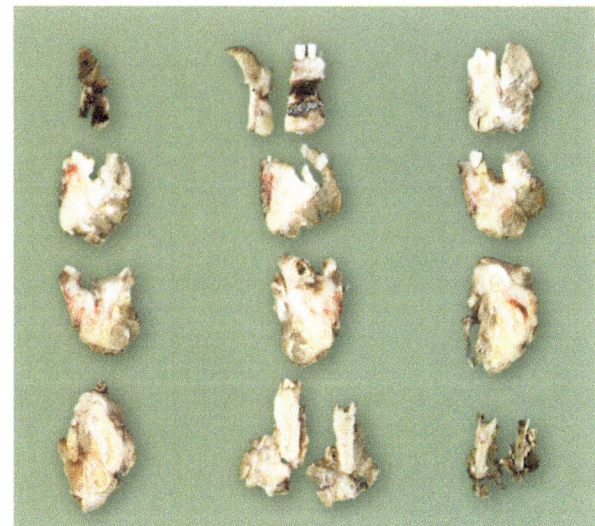

a

b

Figure 2.39
▲

Macroscopic appearance of lingual gingival cancer extending into the adjacent floor of the mouth.

a Occlusal view of specimen showing tumour lingually from the teeth, two of which have gold–porcelain crowns.

b Slices cut in a buccolingual direction visualising tumour at the alveolar process spreading lingually into the floor of the mouth.

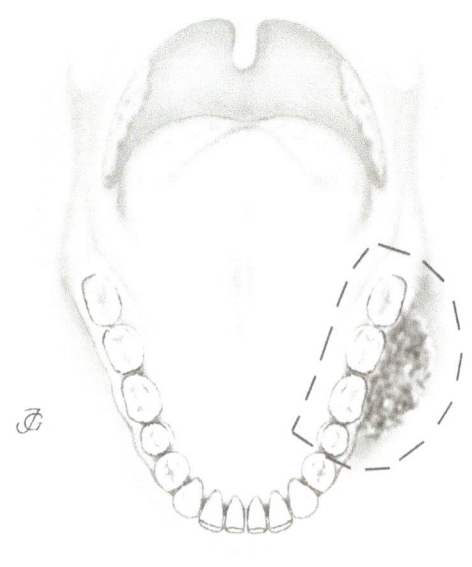

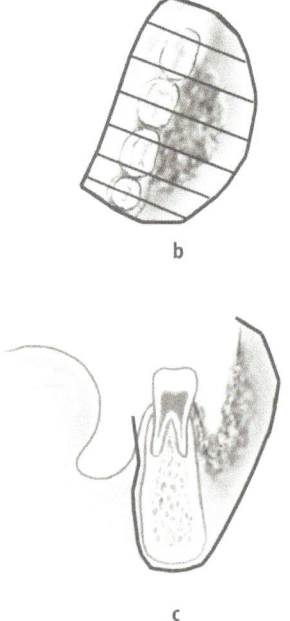

a

b

c

Figure 2..40

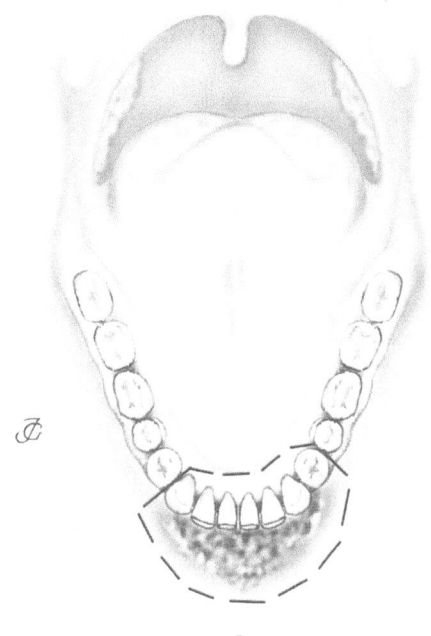

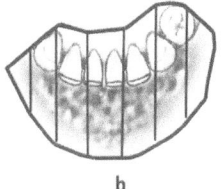

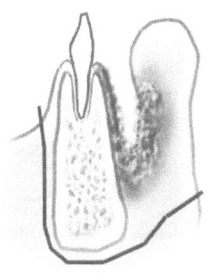

a

b

c

Pathological anatomy of labial gingival cancer spreading into the adjacent lip.

a Clinical appearance and outline of the resection.

b Surgical specimen and plane of sectioning.

c Cut surface showing tumour thickness and involvement of adjacent structures as well as the outline of the resection that includes the lower lip.

Figure 2.41
▲

Pathological anatomy of buccal gingival cancer spreading into the adjacent cheek.

a Clinical appearance and outline of the resection.

b Surgical specimen and plane of sectioning.

c Cut surface showing tumour thickness and involvement of adjacent structures as well as the outline of the resection.

Figure 2.40
◄

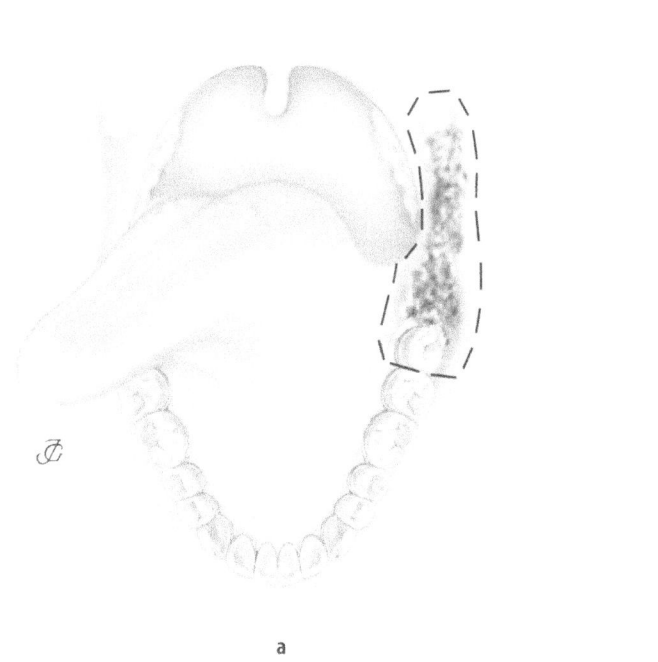

Figure 2.42 ▲

Pathological anatomy of retromolar area cancer.

a Clinical appearance and outline of the resection.

b Surgical specimen and plane of sectioning.

c Cut surface showing relationship with underlying bone.

d Extent of the resection viewed laterally.

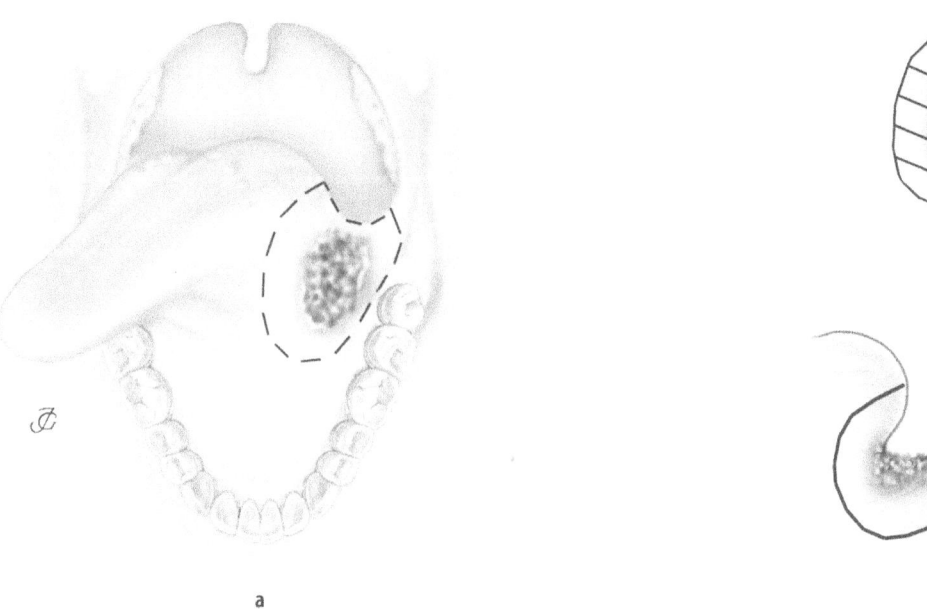

Figure 2.43

These specimens consist of the anterior part of the ascending mandibular ramus with overlying mucosa that may be more or less rectangular. Margins lie at the borders mentioned above under Anatomy.

Dissection

Analysis of these specimens starts with recording the size and site of the lesion, the minimal distance to the resection margin and the location of this closest margin. The best way to dissect these resections is by cutting slices from craniodorsal to caudoventral parallel to the dorsocranial margin, which usually contains the posterior part of the maxillary tuberosity. The cut surface allows measurement of the thickness of the tumour as well as the depth of penetration and reveals whether there is submucosal tumour spread. Also, the minimal distance to the closest deep margin should be recorded, as well as the location of this margin (Fig. 2.42).

Sometimes the lower alveolar nerve lies between mandibular bone and mucosa in this area; its cut surface should be identified at the cranial margin and be sampled for assessment of perineural tumour spread. As the specimen usually contains bone at its deep surface, slicing in this way requires use of the saw. Sometimes only a tiny piece of bone is included within the resection. If there is ample space between tumour and bone this fragment can be removed from the specimen to allow slicing with only a knife. When doing this it is wise to ink the periosteal surface originally covering the removed bony tissue so that, if histological investigation unexpectedly shows tumour to be present in the deep surface, one knows whether this is in the periosteum originally adjacent to bone or in the real deep surface.

Specific Features

Retromolar cancers quite often spread into adjacent mucosal areas, in which case the rules for these adjacent areas also apply. Moreover the retromolar area is often involved by tumour spreading into that area from one of the oropharyngeal sites.

Floor of the Mouth

Anatomy

The floor of the mouth is a horseshoe-shaped mucosal area between the lateral border of the tongue medially and the lingual gingiva of the lower alveolar ridge laterally or, in its anterior part, ventrally. Dorsally, it extends to left and right tonsillar areas.

Anterior in the floor of the mouth, ducts of the bilaterally located submandibular salivary glands open into the oral cavity and cancer at this site may obstruct salivary flow leading to enlargement of these glands that may simulate submandibular lymph node metastasis. Moreover, the tumour may extend along these ducts.

Specimen

Surgical resections from the floor of the mouth are done almost exclusively for treatment of squamous cell carcinoma. Because of the vicinity of the lateral border of the tongue as well as the lingual gingiva of the lower alveolar ridge, lateral and medial resection margins are mostly located in these mucosal areas. Ventral and dorsal margins go through the floor of the mouth; their position is dictated by the tumour size.

Pathological anatomy of cancer of the posterior floor of the mouth.

a Clinical appearance and outline of the resection.

b Surgical specimen and plane of sectioning.

c Cut surface showing relationship of tumour with surrounding structures and outline of the resection.

Figure 2.43
◄

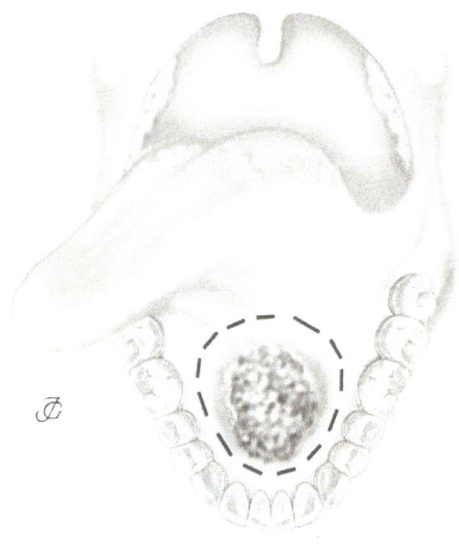

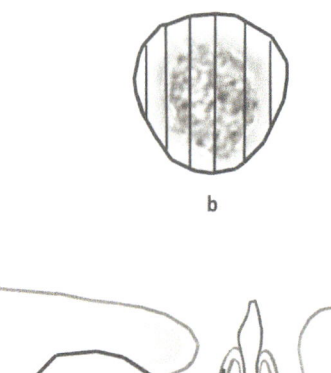

b

a

c

Figure 2.44 ▲	Pathological anatomy of cancer of the anterior floor of mouth.

a Clinical appearance and outline of the resection.

b Surgical specimen and plane of sectioning.

c Cut surface showing relationship of tumour with surrounding structures as well as outline of the resection.

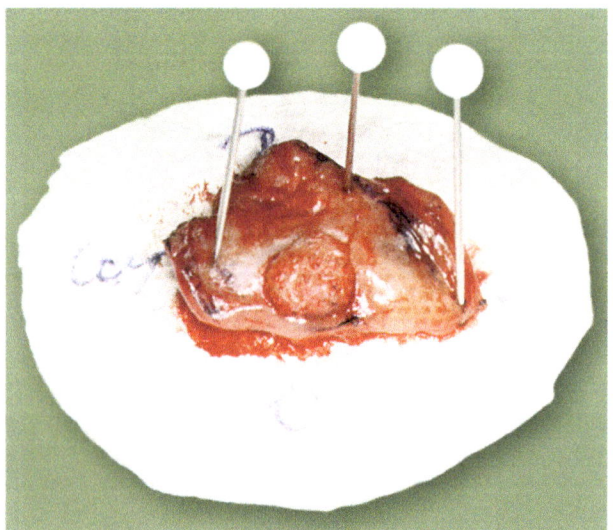

Figure 2.45 ▲	Macroscopic appearance of cancer in the anterior floor of the mouth. If not too large, these tumours can be removed by a limited excision. If these specimens are submitted pinned on a corkboard as shown, accurate sampling of the margins is possible.

Dissection

Examination starts with measuring the size of the mucosal surface, the thickness of the entire specimen as well as the size of the mucosal lesion, its gross appearance, the minimal distance to the closest resection margin and the location of this closest margin. Thereafter the specimen is cut in parallel slices perpendicular to the long axis of the floor of the mouth. In the dorsal part of the floor of the mouth the line of sectioning thus lies in a mediolateral direction; in the anterior part sections are made ventrodorsally (Figs. 2.43–2.45, pages 42–44). To accommodate the curve of the floor of the mouth at the lingual side of the mandibular cuspid area, slices are wedge-shaped, only displaying the lateral or ventral surgical margin (Fig. 2.46, page 46). These sections allow measurement of the lesion's thickness, depth of penetration and involvement of underlying salivary gland tissue, the lingual gland at this location. Moreover the minimal distance between the deep surgical surface and the deep invasion front of the tumour has to be recorded.

Specific Features

In the anterior part of the floor of the mouth the openings of the ducts of the left as well as the right submandibular gland have to be sampled for histological examination to evaluate whether there is intraductal tumour spread. In floor of mouth cancers that spread laterally or ventrally into the alveolar ridge mucosa, the specimens may contain parts of the mandibular bone. In these instances one needs the saw to lengthen the mucosal slices into the bony components. Slicing in this way is necessary to see whether and how the bone is involved by tumour. If floor of mouth cancer spreads medially or dorsally, the tumour involves the lateral border or – in the anterior floor of the mouth – the ventral surface of the mobile tongue. In this case slices are easily lengthened into these soft tissue parts to assess the extent of spread into adjacent anatomical subregions.

Tongue

Anatomy

The tongue is subdivided into the mobile tongue that belongs to the oral cavity and the base of the tongue that belongs to the oropharynx, the line demarcated by the circumvallate papillae separating the two parts. Laterally as well as anteriorly the mucosal surfaces of the mobile tongue merge gradually with the mucosal lining of the floor of the mouth.

Specimen

Tongue resections are done almost exclusively for treatment of squamous cell cancer. Those tumours usually are located at the lateral or ventral border of the tongue and may extend into the adjacent floor of the mouth. Squamous cell cancer of the dorsal surface of the tongue is extremely unusual. The specimens usually consist of a partial glossectomy, its dimensions dictated by the size of the tumour. For tumours located in the more dorsal part of the tongue a hemiglossectomy is usual. More anteriorly located tumours require a near-total glossectomy including the tip of the tongue.

Dissection

Analysis starts with recording the type of glossectomy and the size of the specimen as well as the size, site and appearance of the lesion, minimal distance to the closest resection margin, and the site of this closest margin. Thereafter the specimen is cut in parallel slices perpendicular to the lateral border of the tongue (Figs. 2.47, page 46, 2.48, page 47). Slices thus obtained allow measurement of the lesion's thickness and depth of penetration as well as of the minimal distance between the lesion's deepest invasion front and the deep surgical margin through the tongue musculature. For lesions located more anteriorly, wedge-shaped slices have to be made to follow the curve of the tongue where it goes from lateral border to tip (Fig. 2.49, page 47).

Specific Features

In the case of tongue tumours that extend into the floor of the mouth the slices will also contain these adjacent mucosal parts. In the case of tongue tumours extending not only into the floor of the mouth but also into adjacent alveolar ridge the slices will also contain parts of the mandibular bone as mentioned in the Floor of the Mouth section. These

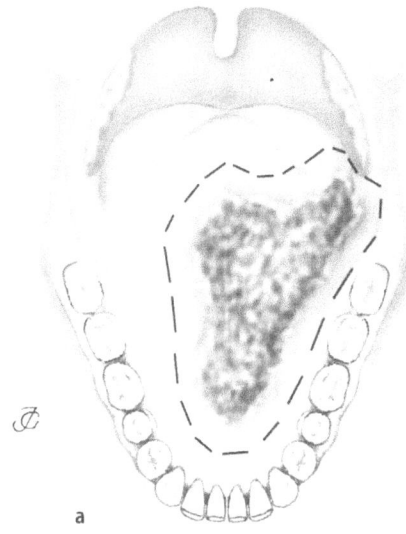

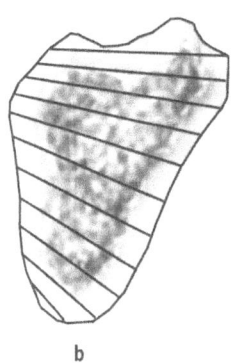

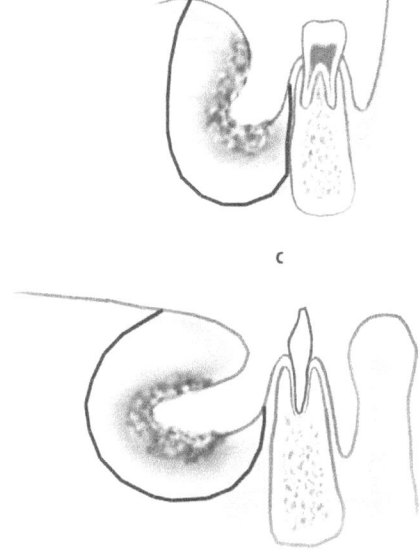

Figure 2.46 Pathological anatomy of cancer involving the anterior as well as the posterior floor of the mouth.

a Clinical appearance and outline of the resection.

b Surgical specimen and plane of sectioning, which rotates slightly from buccolingual posteriorly to dorsoventral anteriorly to accommodate the curve of the floor of the mouth.

c Cut surface showing tumour extension, outline of the resection, and relationship with surroundings posteriorly.

d Cut surface showing tumour extension, outline of the resection, and relationship with surroundings anteriorly.

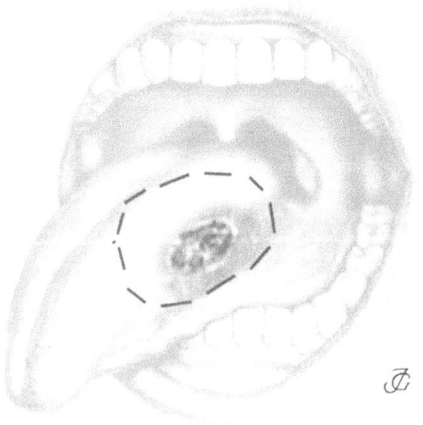

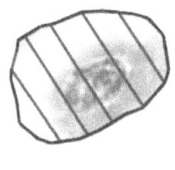

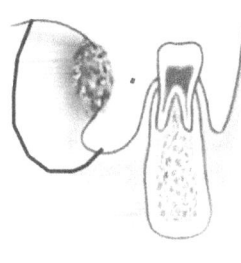

Figure 2.47 Pathological anatomy of cancer at the lateral border of the tongue.

a Clinical appearance and outline of the resection.

b Surgical specimen and plane of sectioning.

c Cut surface showing position and extension of tumour as well as the outline of the resection.

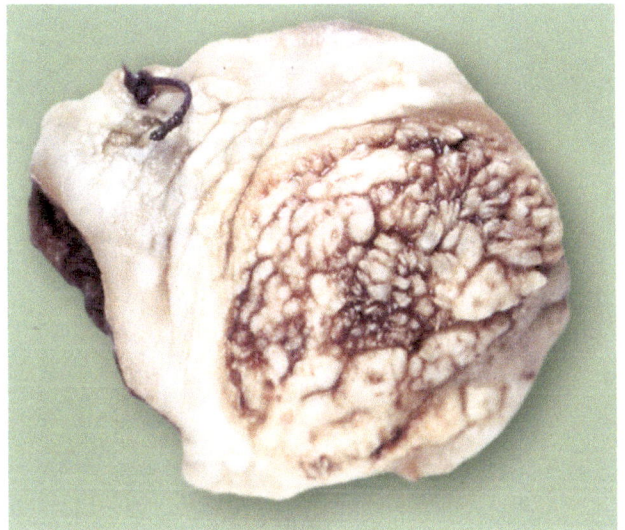
a

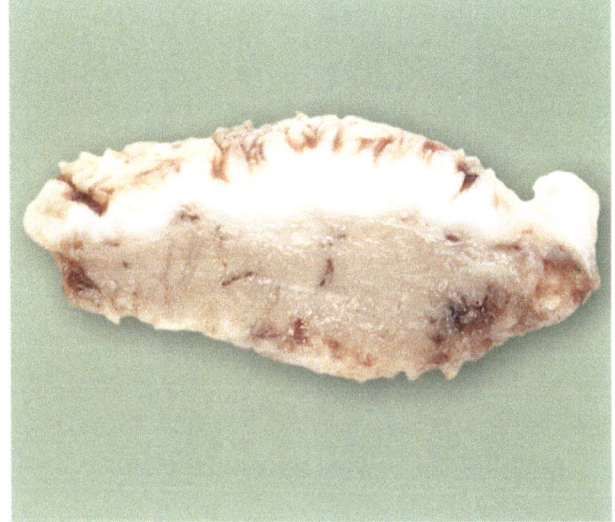
b

Macroscopic appearance of cancer at the lateral border of the tongue.

a Surgical specimen.

b Cut surface.

Figure 2.48
▲

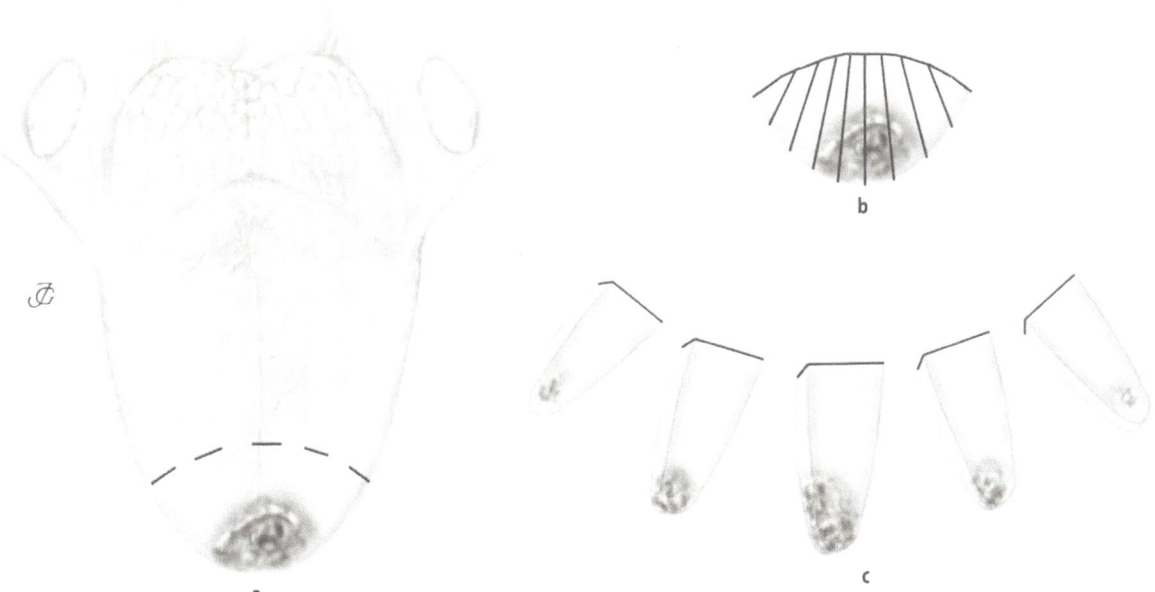

Pathological anatomy of cancer at the tip of the tongue.

a Clinical appearance and outline of the resection.

b Surgical specimen and plane of sectioning, which rotates to remain perpendicular to the free margin of the tongue.

c Slices obtained when sectioning perpendicular to the free edge of the tongue tip and lateral border.

Figure 2.49
▲

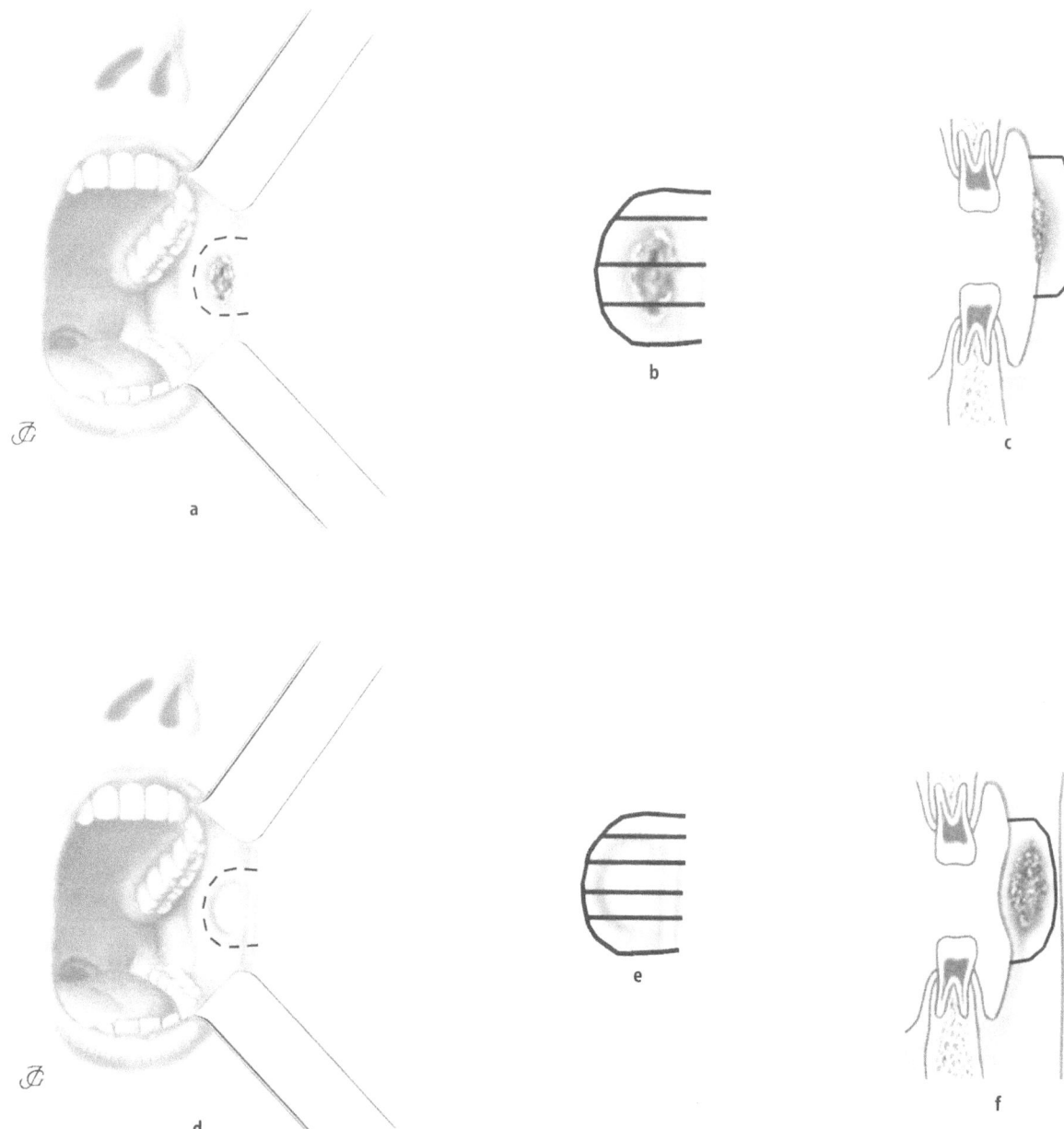

b

Figure 2.50
▲

Pathological anatomy of tumours in the cheek.

a–c Mucosal cancer.

a Clinical appearance and outline of the resection.

b Surgical specimen and plane of sectioning.

c Cut surface showing tumour position and relationship with adjacent structures as well as the outline of the resection.

d–f Submucosal cheek tumour.

d Clinical appearance and outline of the resection.

e Surgical specimen and plane of sectioning.

f Cut surface showing tumour covered with an uninvolved mucosal layer, as well as the outline of the resection.

specimens are dissected in accordance with the guidelines for cancers of the lingual mandibular gingiva extending into the floor of the mouth and lateral border of tongue.

In the case of dorsally located tongue tumours, one should identify and sample the margin through the lingual nerve for analysis of perineural tumour spread into this surgical margin. This nerve can be found at the dorsolateral surgical margin.

Cheek

Anatomy

The cheek is covered by the buccal mucosa, which extends from the retromolar trigone posteriorly to the lips anteriorly. Its upper and lower borders are formed by the junction with the upper and lower oral vestibule.

Specimen

Cheek resections are done for squamous cell carcinoma or submucosally located salivary gland tumours. Mostly they consist of a more or less rectangular piece of tissue covered with a mucosal lining, the deep surface being composed of muscular tissue or fatty tissue. Only in the case of deeply penetrating tumours is a full-thickness resection done, resulting in a specimen with an inner mucosal and an outer skin covering.

Dissection

Analysis begins with inspection and measuring. One should note whether the lesion is mucosal or sub-

mucosal and, in the latter case, should record whether the lesion is covered with an uninvolved freely mobile mucosal lining or whether there is penetration of the lesion through the mucosal lining. In the case of a mucosal lesion one should note its appearance and measure its size as well as the minimal distance to the closest resection margin and the site of this closest margin. Thereafter the specimen should be sliced in a horizontal plane. Slices thus obtained allow – in the case of a mucosal lesion – measurement of the thickness of the lesion, depth of penetration and minimal distance to the deep margins (Figs. 2.50, page 48, 2.51, page 50).

In the case of a submucosal lesion such as a salivary gland lesion, these slices allow determination of the lesion's maximal size, its outline and the minimal distance to the resection margin as well as the site of this margin. Moreover these slices display which structures are involved by tumour: fatty submucosal tissue, muscle tissue, or both.

Specific Features

Tumours may extend ventrally into the corner of the mouth. Horizontal slicing allows inspection of the transition between mucosa and skin at this site. Sometimes a cheek tumour may spread beyond the corner of the mouth. In that case the rules for lip dissection apply for that part of the specimen, as discussed under Lip above. Tumours may also extend into the upper or lower vestibular fold and involve the buccal side of the alveolar ridge. In these cases cheek resections may contain a rim of either mandibular or maxillary bone. In that event the specimen should be dissected according to the guidelines given for cancers of mandibular or maxillary buccal gingiva extending across the vestibular fold into the cheek.

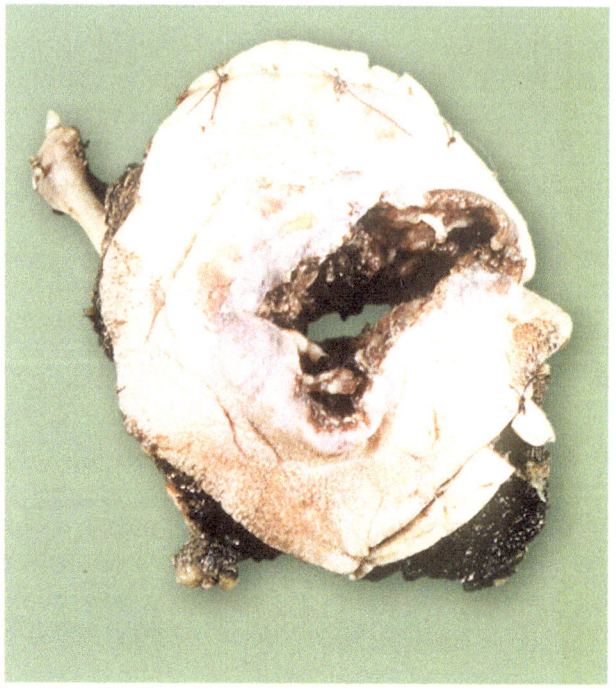

a

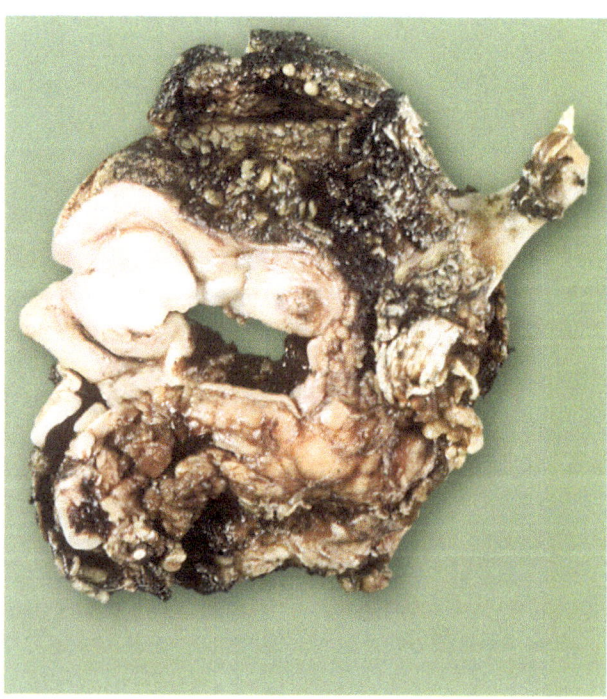

b

Figure 2.51
▲

Macroscopic appearance of cheek tumour penetrating into the skin.

a Lateral view showing skin defect.

b Medial view showing mucosal surface. The size of the tumour made removal of the mandible also necessary.

Oropharynx 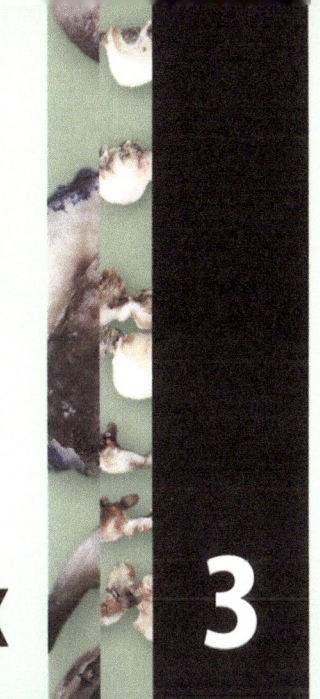 3

General Remarks

The oropharynx forms part of the pharynx, a hollow tube that extends from the base of the skull cranially to the lower border of the cricoid cartilage caudally. Cranially, the oropharynx merges with the nasopharynx, the border between the two being at the level of the hard palate; the lower border lies at the horizontal plane through the vallecula where the oropharynx is continuous with the hypopharynx. The oropharynx has anterior, lateral, posterior and superior walls. The anterior wall is formed by the base of the tongue and the vallecula. The lateral walls are the tonsils, the faucial pillars and the glossotonsillar sulci. The superior wall is represented by the inferior surface of the soft palate and the uvula, and the posterior wall lies anteriorly to the second and third cervical vertebrae. Anterior, lateral and inferior walls line the isthmus through which the oropharynx opens into the oral cavity. Specimens may come from each of the oropharyngeal walls.

Base of the Tongue

Anatomy

A line demarcated by the circumvallate papillae separates the base of the tongue from the mobile tongue. Posteriorly the base of the tongue ends in the vallecula, which forms the border with the base of the epiglottis. The lateral borders are the glossotonsillar sulci that separate the base of the tongue from the tonsils and the tonsillar fossae as well as the faucial pillars.

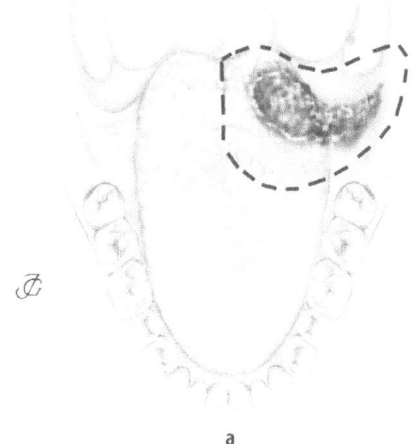

a

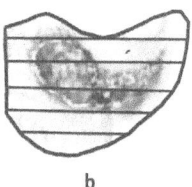

b

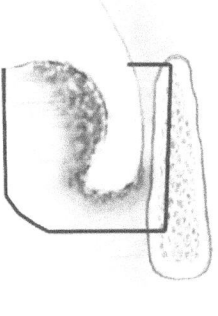

c

Figure 3.1   Pathological anatomy of tumour at the lateral base of the tongue.

a Clinical appearance and outline of the resection.

b Surgical specimen and plane of sectioning.

c Cut surface exhibiting relationship of tumour to surroundings including mandibular bone as well as the outline of the resection.

Specimen

Resections that contain parts of the base of the tongue are usually performed to treat squamous cell cancer, less often to remove submucosally lying salivary gland tumours. Mostly these specimens also contain adjacent areas from the oropharynx or parts from the oral cavity or the larynx. Which adjacent anatomical subsites are included within the resection depends on the site of the lesion. Tumours located laterally may spread into the retromolar trigone, anterior faucial pillar and tonsil. Medially situated tumours invade the extrinsic tongue musculature and may extend posteriorly to the epiglottis and pre-epiglottic space.

Dissection

The specimen usually consists of muscular tissue with adjacent loose fibro-fatty tissue containing accessory salivary glands and covered with a mucosal lining. Examination starts with determining the size and site of the mucosal lesion, the minimal distance to the resection margin, and the location of this closest margin. Thereafter the specimen is cut in slices parallel to the anterior margin, which usually goes through the mobile tongue just anterior to the circumvallate papillae (Fig. 3.1). These slices allow assessment of tumour thickness as well as depth of penetration. Moreover the minimal distance between the deep tumour front and the deep resection margins has to be determined. These specimens have deep margins dorsally facing the pre-epiglottic space, and anteriorly as well as medially going through the muscular tissue of the tongue.

Specific Features

Tumours of the tongue may spread laterally into the retromolar area or tonsillar fossa. In those instances the parallel slices are lengthened into these adjacent areas. In addition there may be dorsal spread into the pre-epiglottic space, in which case these tumours in spite of having originated in the base of the tongue may resemble supraglottic cancers that have spread anteriorly into the base of the tongue (Figs. 3.2, page 54, 3.3, page 55). In this instance, surgical treatment consists of removing the base of the tongue as well as the larynx. Dissection of these specimens is done in the same way as for supraglottic cancers and will be discussed in Chapter 4.

Soft Palate

Anatomy

The soft palate represents a mucosal fold with a core consisting of fibrous and muscular tissue and containing fatty and salivary gland tissue. Anteriorly it has a junction with the hard palate. Laterally it merges with the cranial part of the tonsillar fossa, and dorsally it has a free margin where oral and nasal surface meet and that is separated into two halves by the uvula. Tumours in this area may spread into the tonsillar fossa laterally or may cross the midline medially.

Specimen

Parts of the soft palate are usually resected for treatment of squamous cell cancer originating in the epithelium lining its oral surface, or to remove salivary gland tumours originating within the deeper palatal tissue layers. There are basically two types of resections: those including the free dorsal margin and those in which the dorsal margin has been saved.

Dissection

Irrespective of whether the specimen includes the free palatal margin or not, examination begins with recording whether there is a mucosal lesion and, if so, its site, size, minimal distance to the resection margin, and the location of this closest margin. In the case of submucosally located lesions the size of the lesion is determined by palpation and it is noted whether there is perforation of this lesion through either oral or nasal mucosal surface. When the specimen includes the free margin it is cut in parallel slices perpendicular to this free margin (Fig. 3.4, page 56). When the specimen only contains the more

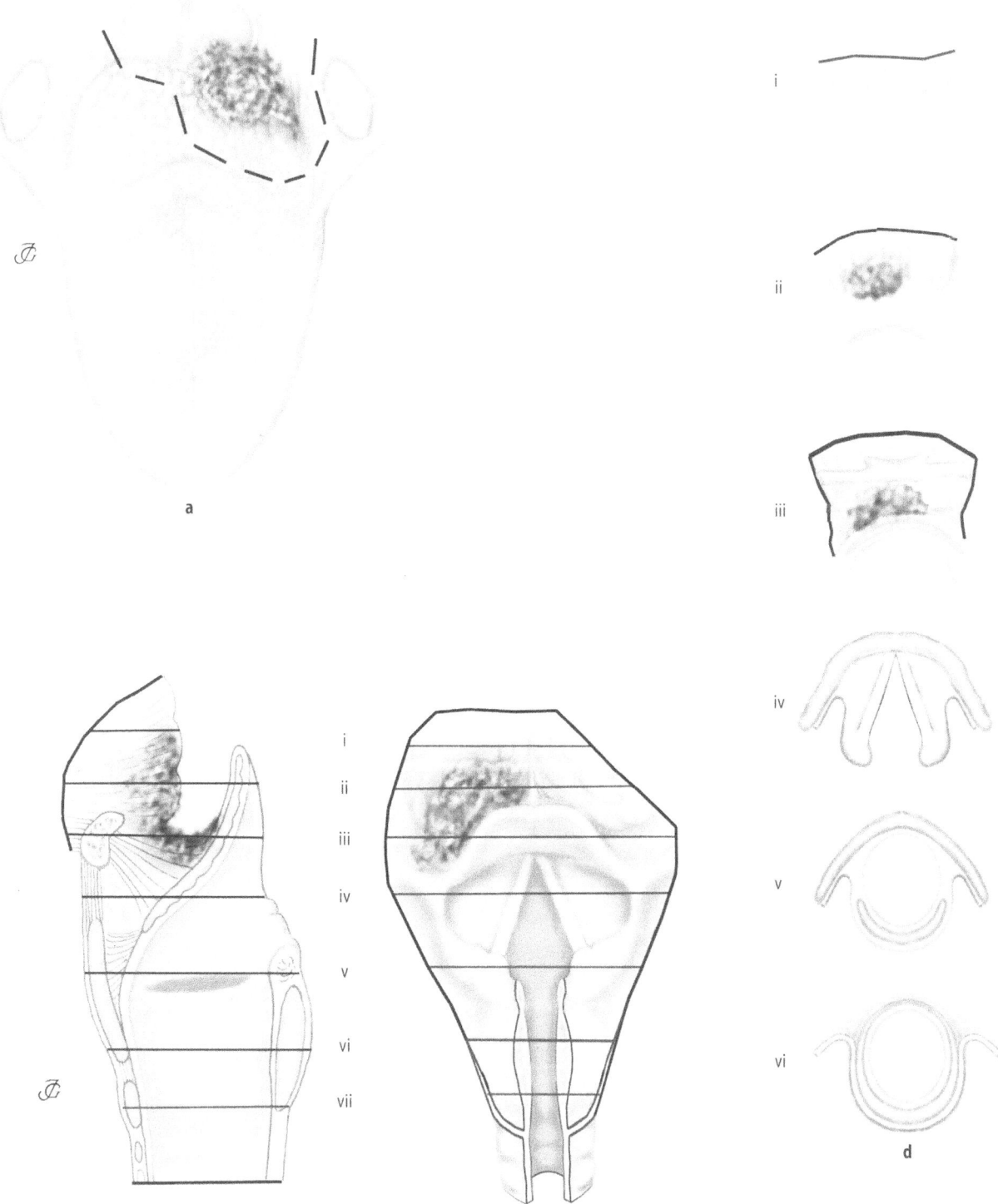

Figure 3.2

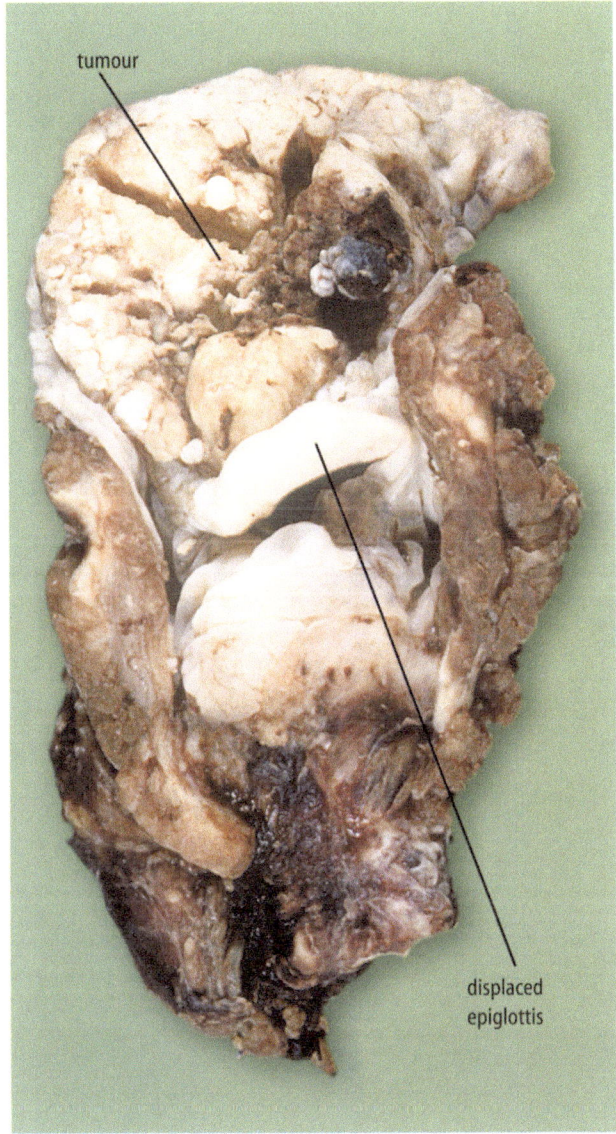

tumour

displaced
epiglottis

a

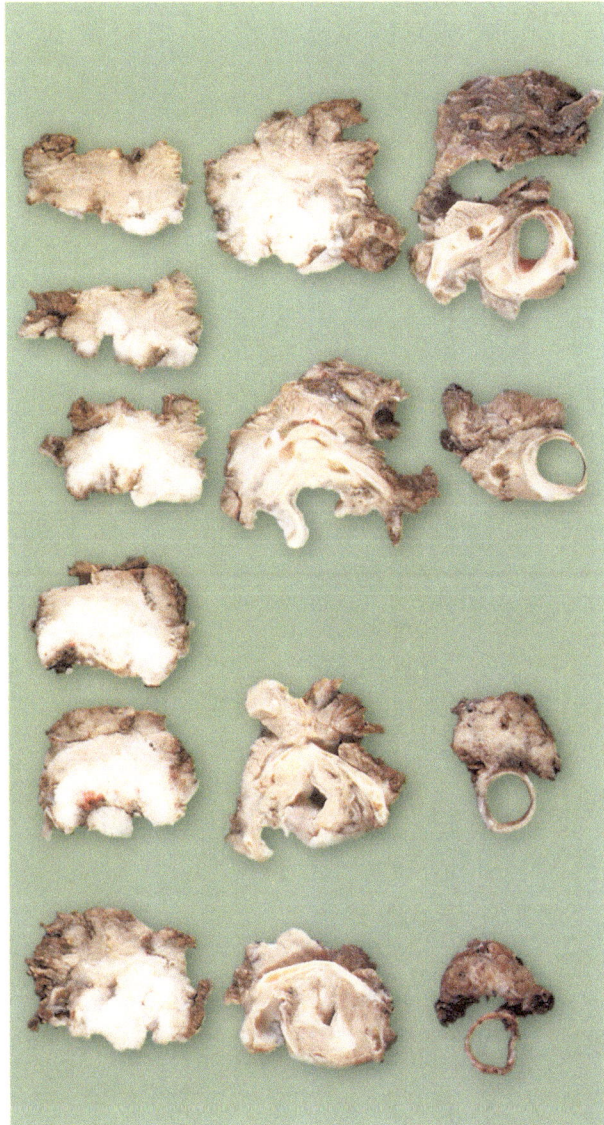

b

Macroscopic appearance of vallecular cancer.

a Posterior view showing tumour in the vallecula causing posterior displacement of the epiglottis.

b Slices obtained when cutting the specimen horizontally from cranial to caudal, displaying tumour size and extension.

Figure 3.3
▲

Pathological anatomy of tumour at the vallecula.

a Superior view showing clinical appearance and outline of the resection. These specimens also contain the larynx.

b Sagittal cut surface showing tumour extension anteriorly into the base of the tongue and posteriorly involving the epiglottis. Horizontal lines i–vii indicate planes of sectioning. Ventrally, a line is drawn to indicate the anterior surgical margin.

c Surgical specimen and planes of sectioning i–vii viewed from dorsally.

d Slices i–vi obtained when cutting the specimen as indicated in **b** and **c**.

Figure 3.2
◄

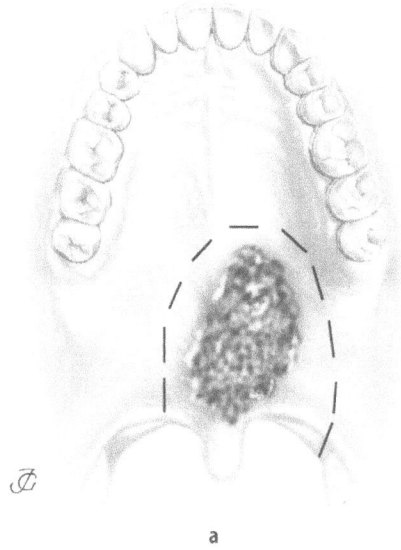

a

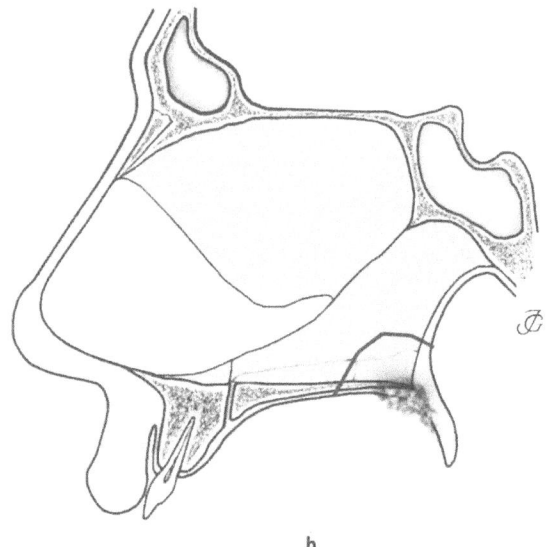

b

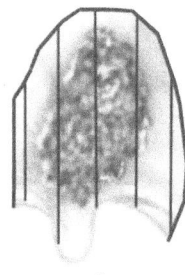

c

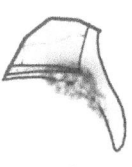

d

Figure 3.4
▲

Pathological anatomy of mucosal cancer at the soft palate.

a Clinical appearance and outline of the resection.

b Sagittal view showing the tumour in relation to surrounding structures and outline of the resection.

c Surgical specimen and plane of sectioning.

d Cut surface showing tumour thickness and relationship with adjacent palatal structures.

anterior part of the soft palate then it is cut in parallel slices in a mediolateral direction parallel to either the anterior or the posterior surgical margin (Fig. 3.5, page 58). In both instances slices thus obtained should be examined for tumour thickness as well as depth of penetration for mucosal cancer, and for maximal size and involvement of palatal structures when dealing with salivary gland tumours.

Specific Features

If there is tumour extension laterally into the tonsillar area, the plane of sectioning will rotate from ventrodorsally to mediolaterally to accommodate the arching of the faucial pillars. These slices will display the dorsolateral resection margin through the pharyngeal musculature (Figs. 3.6, page 58, 3.7, page 60).

Tonsillar Area

Anatomy

The tonsillar area is bordered by the anterior and posterior faucial pillar and ventrally by the base of the tongue, from which it is separated by the glossotonsillar sulci. Cranially this area is continuous with the inferior surface of the soft palate.

Specimen

Tumours in this usually area are squamous cell cancers arising in the mucosal lining. They may involve the faucial pillars as well as the tonsillar area proper. In the latter case they are sometimes located in a tonsillar crypt without causing any mucosal abnormality and thus difficult to visualise macroscopically. Tonsillar squamous cell cancer may extend into adjacent areas belonging to other parts of the oropharynx or forming part of the oral cavity.

Dissection

The specimen usually consists of the tonsillar fossa proper together with parts of adjacent regions: the

base of the tongue medioventrally, the retromolar trigone lateroventrally and the soft palate mediocranially. Examination begins with recording the size and site of the lesion, minimal distance to the resection margin, and the location of this closest margin.

Thereafter, the specimen is cut in slices parallel to the dorsocranial margin, going from craniodorsal to caudoventral (Figs. 3.8, page 61, 3.9, page 62). When examining these slices one should realise that the presence of tonsillar tissue seriously hampers evaluation of tumour thickness as well as depth of penetration, as the firm and white tonsillar tissue closely mimics invading squamous cell cancer. Therefore it is prudent to process all slices containing tonsillar tissue for paraffin embedding and histological examination, not only to be able to discriminate between tonsillar tissue and invading tumour but also to analyse whether there is tumour involving tonsillar crypts that is not visible with the naked eye.

Specific Features

In the case of spread of tonsillar cancer into adjacent areas the plane of sectioning does not change. Slices are lengthened into these areas. If the tumour spreads from the tonsillar area into the soft palate, including its free margin, then the guidelines given for cancer of the soft palate extending into the tonsillar fossa apply.

Posterior Pharyngeal Wall

Anatomy

The superior border of the oropharyngeal part of the posterior pharyngeal wall is at the level of the soft palate; the lower border is at the level of the vallecula. Anteriorly the posterior pharyngeal wall merges with the medial faucial pillar. Dorsally lies the prevertebral fascia.

Specimen

Resections of the posterior pharyngeal wall are done for treatment of squamous cell cancer. These tumours may extend cranially into the nasopharynx,

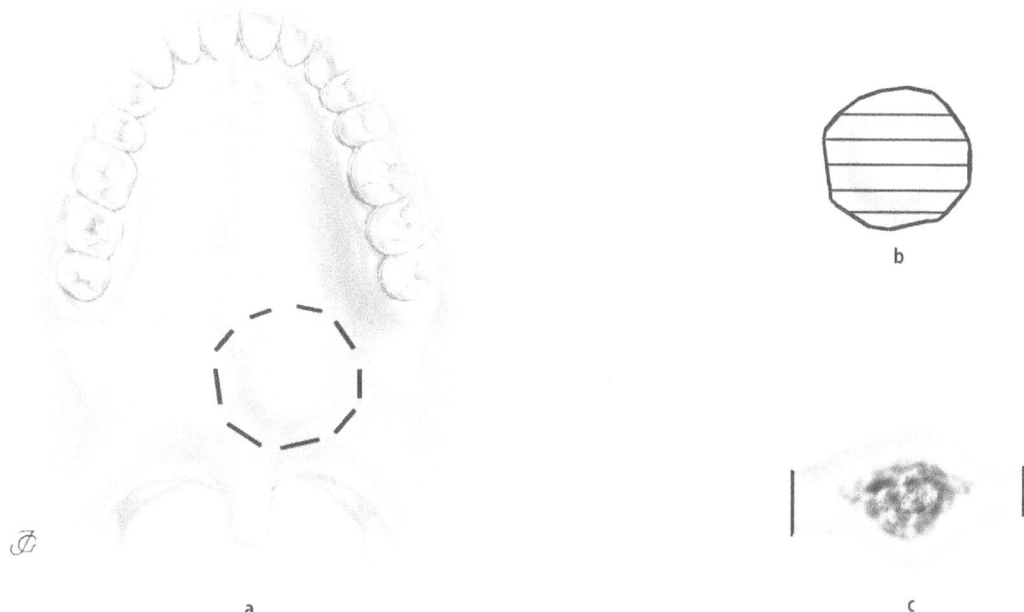

a

c

b

Figure 3.5
▲

Pathological anatomy of submucosal tumour at the soft palate.

a Clinical appearance and outline of the resection.

b Surgical specimen and plane of sectioning.

c Cut surface showing tumour located submucosally.

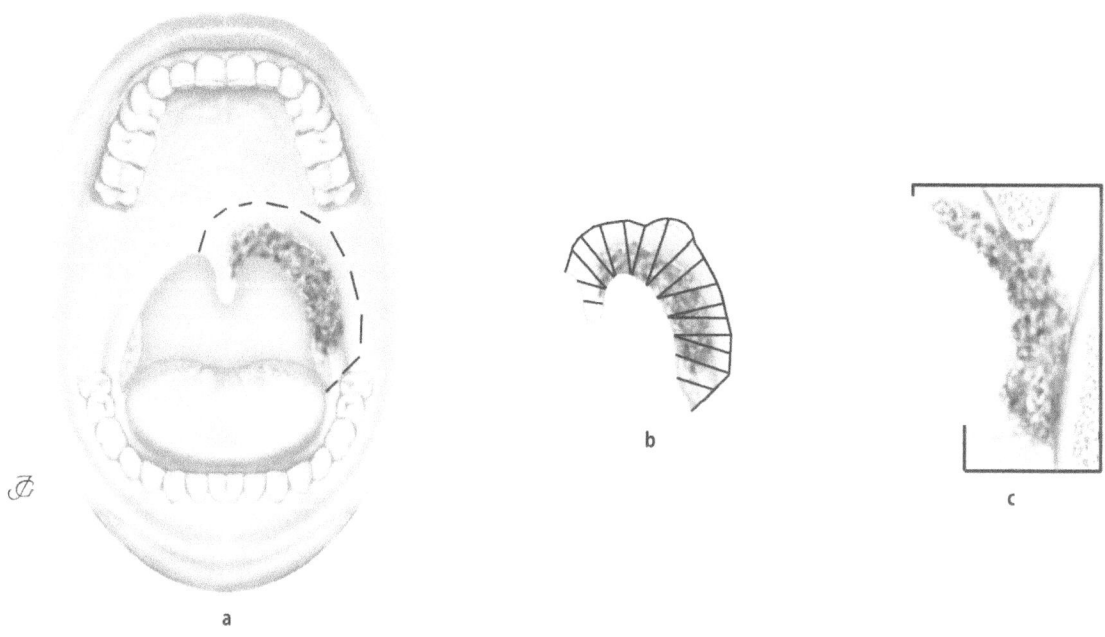

a

b

c

Figure 3.6

posteriorly into the prevertebral fascia, anteriorly into the tonsillar area and soft palate, and caudally into hypopharynx and pyriform sinuses.

Dissection

Usually the specimen is more or less rectangular and consists of muscular tissue and with a mucosal surface. If there is tumour spread into adjacent areas, they are included within the resection. As resections of the posterior pharyngeal wall are done to treat squamous cell cancer, examination will begin with noting the size of the lesion, the minimal distance to the surgical margin, and the location of this closest margin. Thereafter the specimen is cut in slices parallel to the cranial surgical margin and

slices thus obtained allow assessment of the lesion's thickness, depth of penetration, and minimal distance between the tumour front and deep muscular resection margin (Fig. 3.10, page 63).

Specific Features

If there is tumour spread anteriorly into the faucial arch, horizontally cut slices will include this part of the specimen. If the tumour extends into the posterior wall of the hypopharynx, horizontal slices will also be made through this part of the specimen. If the tumour extends into the pyriform sinus, then the guidelines for hypopharyngeal–pyriform sinus cancer have to be followed; these will be dealt with in Chapter 4 (p. 71).

Pathological anatomy of tumour at the soft palate extending laterally into adjacent tonsillar area.

Figure 3.6
◄

a Clinical appearance and outline of the resection.

b Surgical specimen and plane of sectioning. The plane of sectioning rotates to accommodate the curved axis of the specimen.

c Cut surface showing relationship with bone of the maxillary tuberosity and mandible that both may form part of these specimens.

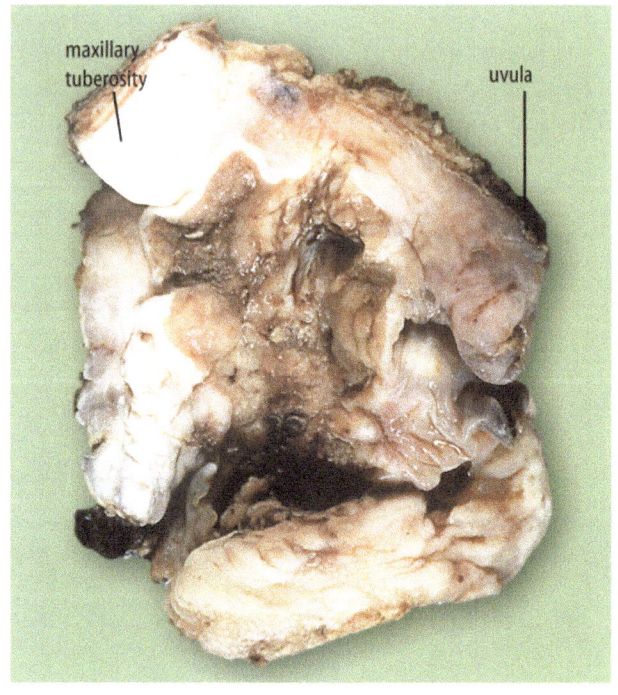

a

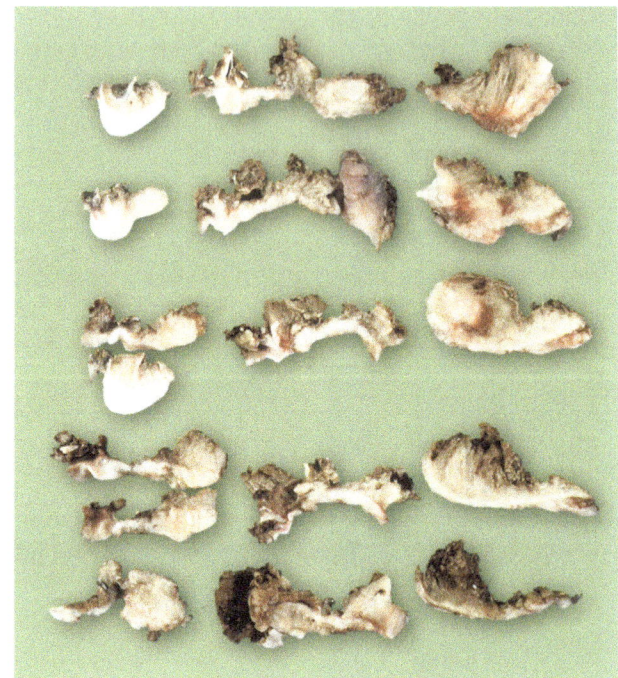

b

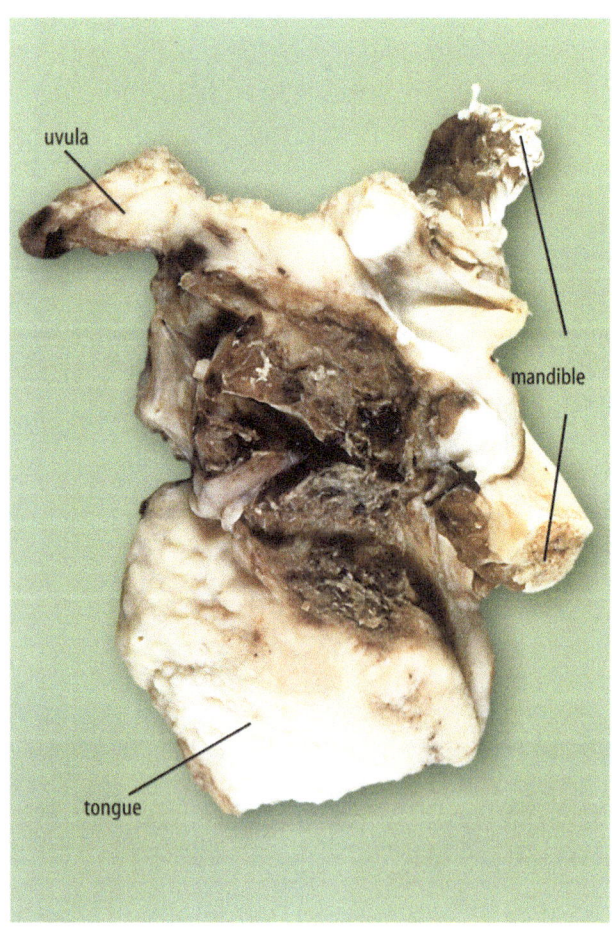

c

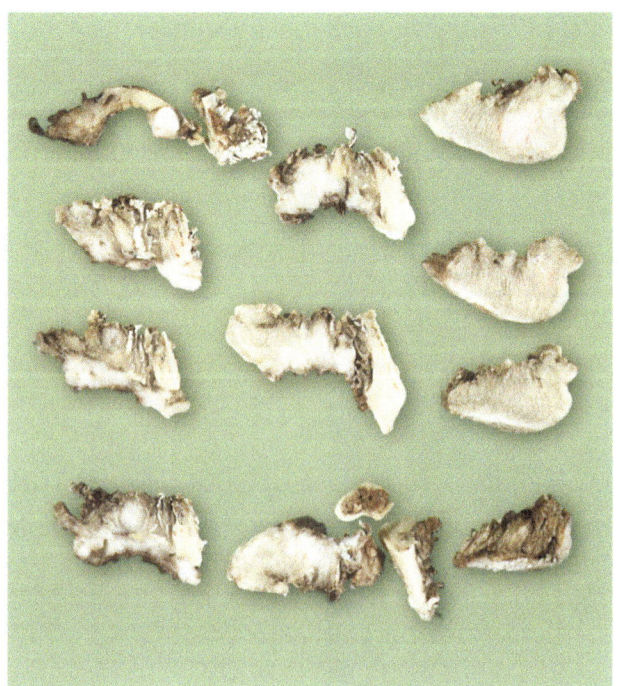

d

Figure 3.7

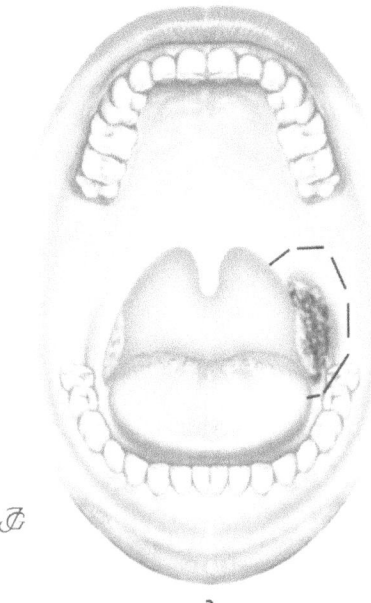

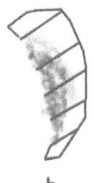

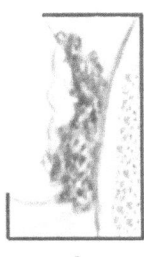

Pathological anatomy of cancer at the tonsillar fossa.

a Clinical appearance and outline of the resection.

b Surgical specimen and plane of sectioning.

c Cut surface showing relationship of tumour with adjacent mandibular bone.

Figure 3.8
▲

Macroscopic appearances of oropharyngeal cancers.

a Tumour in the soft palate between the uvula and maxillary tuberosity.

b Same specimen sectioned as shown in Fig. 3.6.

c Tumour in the soft palate spreading into the base of the tongue and the retromolar area thus necessitating partial removal of the mandible.

d Same specimen sectioned as shown in Fig. 3.6.

Figure 3.7
◄

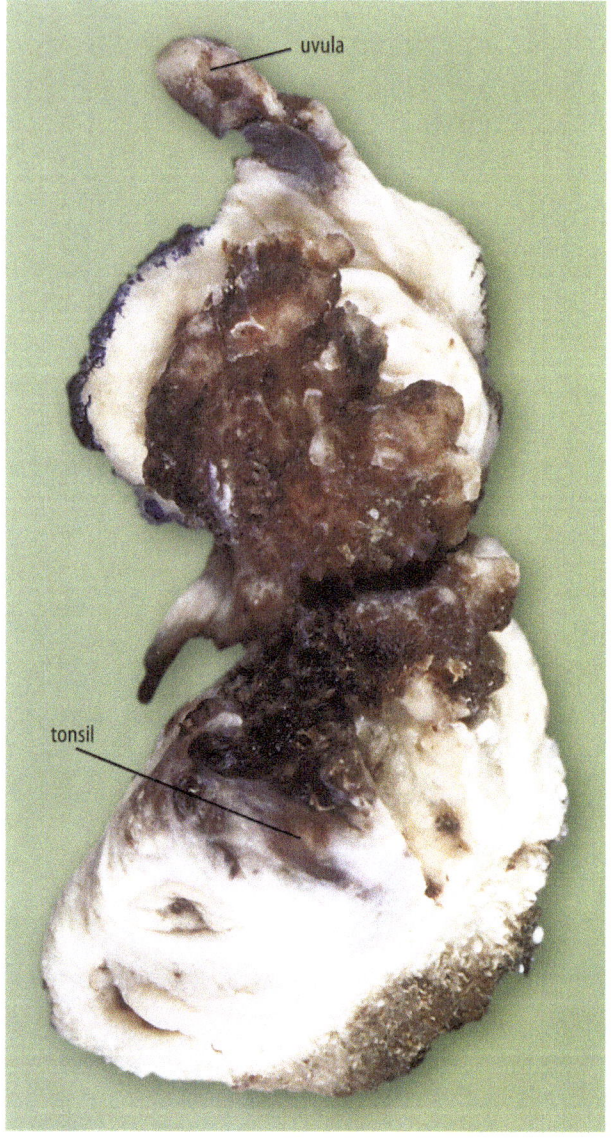

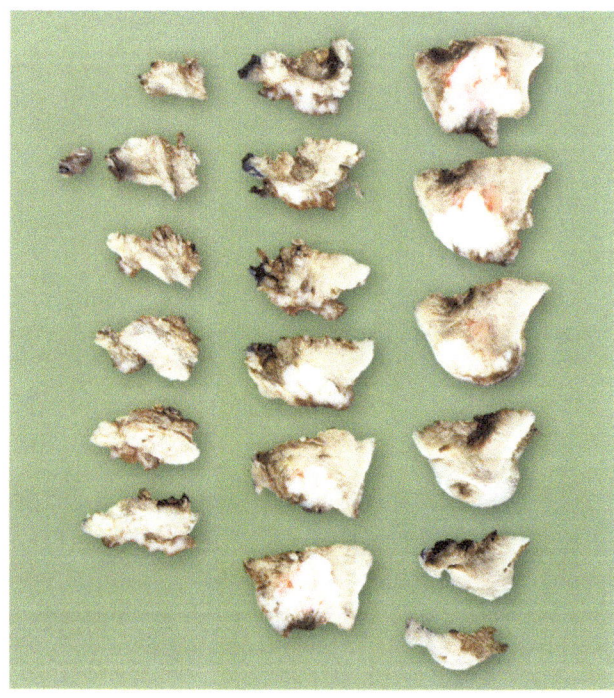

a

b

Figure 3.9
▲

a Macroscopic appearance of cancer of the soft palate spreading into the tonsillar area.

b Slices obtained when sectioning the specimen as shown in Fig. 3.8.

Figure 3.10
▶

Pathological anatomy of tumour at the posterior pharyngeal wall.

a Clinical appearance and outline of the resection. The mandible and tongue are split sagittally to allow visualisation of tumour at this site.

b Sagittal view to display the position of the tumour in relation to surrounding structures, as well as the outline of the resection.

c Surgical specimen and plane of sectioning.

d Cut surface showing tumour spread and thickness.

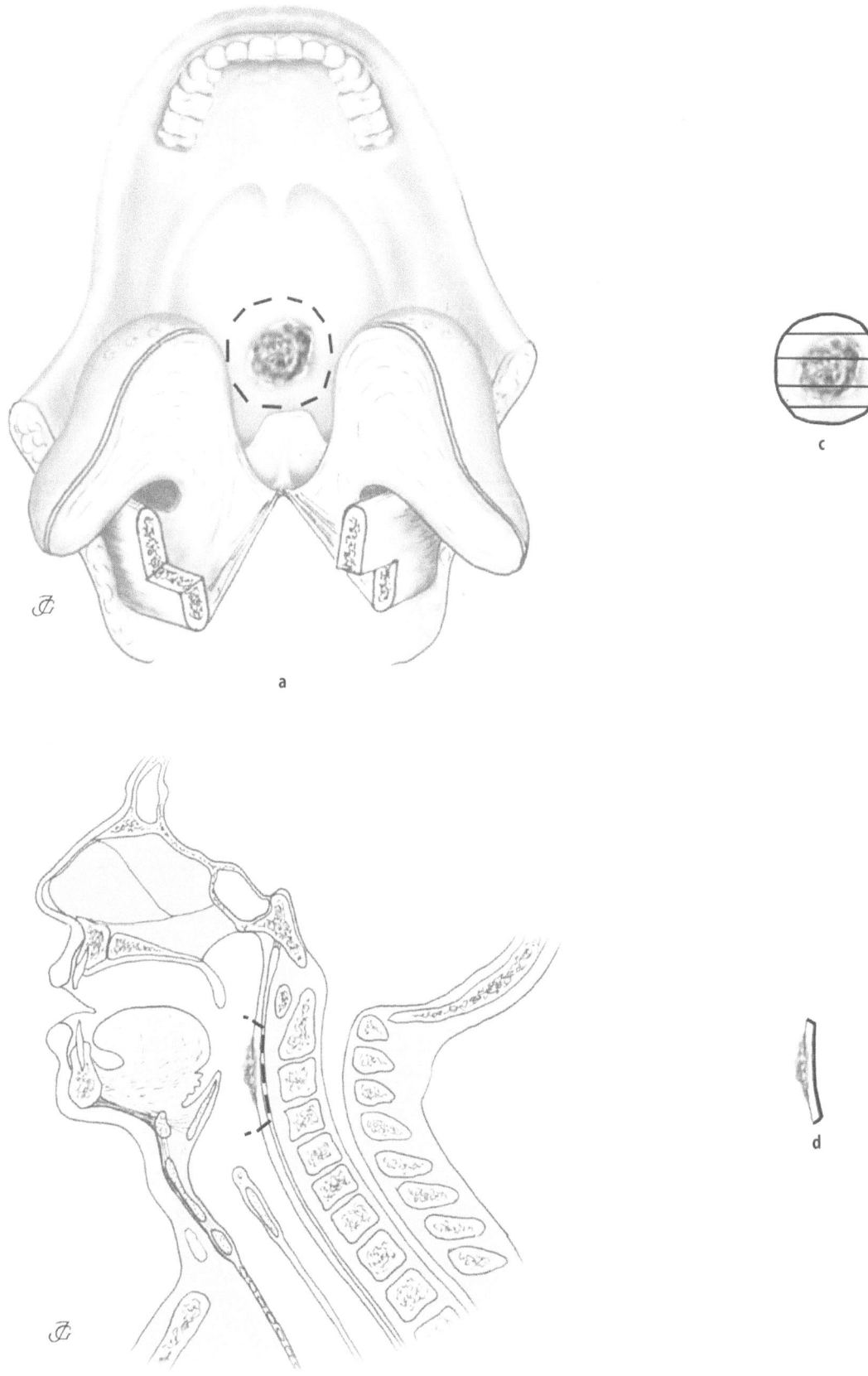

a

c

b

d

Figure 3.10

Larynx and Hypopharynx

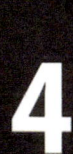

4

General Remarks

The hypopharynx and larynx are anatomically intimately associated and constitute the division point between the digestive tract and lower respiratory tract. Because of their close anatomical relationship, we will discuss the features regarding specimen and dissection for hypopharynx and larynx together. Before this we will discuss the anatomical features of each region separately.

Hypopharynx

Anatomy

The hypopharynx is the most caudal part of the pharynx. It communicates superiorly with the oropharynx and inferiorly with the larynx and oesophagus. The superior border of the hypopharynx is an imaginary horizontal line at the level of the vallecula. The inferior boundary is anteriorly formed by the aryepiglottic folds that separate the hypopharynx from the larynx and posteriorly by the inlet to the oesophagus.

Specific subsites within the hypopharynx are the left and right pyriform sinus and the postcricoid region. The pyriform sinuses are elongated pear-shaped, three-walled gutters that open medially into the hypopharyngeal cavity and extend anterior and laterally on either side of the larynx. The lateral wall of the pyriform sinus covers the medial side of the thyroid cartilage and blends into the posterior pharyngeal wall. Inferiorly the pyriform sinus is in continuity with the postcricoid region, a funnel-shaped area extending from the posterior

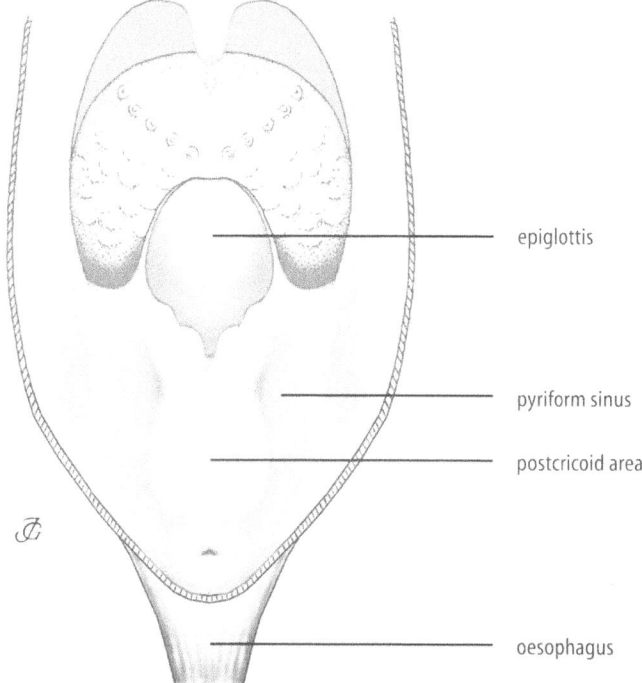

epiglottis

pyriform sinus

postcricoid area

oesophagus

Figure 4.1   Posterior view of the laryngeal entrance with surroundings.

surface of the arytenoid cartilage to the inferior surface of the cricoid cartilage and ending where the oesophagus begins (Fig. 4.1).

Larynx

Anatomy

The larynx is divided into three subsites: supraglottic, glottic and subglottic regions. The supraglottic area extends from the tip of the epiglottis superiorly to the ventricle inferiorly. Encompassed within the supraglottic area are the epiglottis (lingual and laryngeal aspects), the laryngeal aspect of the aryepiglottic folds, the arytenoids, the false vocal cords, and the ventricles. The pre-epiglottic space lies anterior to the epiglottis. The inferior border of the supraglottis is an imaginary horizontal line across the apex of the ventricle. The glottis includes the paired true vocal cords and the anterior and posterior commissure. The inferior border of the glottic area is 1 cm below the apex of the ventricle. The subglottic area extends from the lower edge of the glottis to the inferior aspect of the cricoid cartilage.

Specimen

Surgical treatment of tumours – in most instances squamous cell cancers – in either larynx or hypopharynx usually necessitates removal of the entire larynx as well as parts of the hypopharynx. These tumours may have originated in the hypopharynx with subsequent spread into the laryngeal structures or vice versa.

Laryngohypopharyngectomies consist of a hollow tube, the larynx, that opens cranially into a mucosal surface. Anteriorly this mucosal surface lines the vallecula and the lingual surface of the epiglottis; laterally it covers the pyriform sinus; and posteriorly it forms the anterior wall of the postcricoid area of the hypopharynx. In this way a mucosal surface is formed that slopes from ventrocranial to dorsocaudal, thus making an acute angle with the long axis of the larynx proper and having a ventrocranial, a dorsocaudal and two laterovertical surgical margins.

Cranially, a laryngohypopharyngectomy specimen may be extended by including parts of the base of the tongue in the case of cranially located pyriform sinus cancers or supraglottic cancers. Caudally, dependent on the tumour site, the specimen may contain a varying number of tracheal rings. If a tracheostoma has been made beforehand, this usually is removed together with the larynx. For pyriform sinus cancers the homolateral half of the thyroid gland forms part of the surgical specimen. In selected cases a partial laryngectomy is done; in this procedure either the supraglottic larynx or the left or right lateral laryngeal halves form the specimen.

The larynx may arrive in the pathology laboratory either still as a closed tube or already opened by the surgeon through a vertical dorsal incision allowing visualisation of the endolaryngeal mucosal surface (Fig. 4.2, page 68).

The size of the hypopharyngeal mucosal surface included within a laryngohypopharyngectomy will depend on the site of the tumour. In the case of endolaryngeal cancers the specimen will contain only a narrow strip of hypopharyngeal mucosa, whereas in the case of laryngectomies done for hypopharyngeal cancer more extensive areas of the hypopharyngeal walls are included within the resection (Fig. 4.3, page 69).

Dissection

Investigation of these specimens starts with determination of the site of the tumour as well its size. For the endolarynx all anatomical structures involved by the tumour are identified. This means recording whether the tumour is supraglottic, glottic or subglottic. Supraglottic tumours involve the false vocal cords, the ventricle and the epiglottis (laryngeal or lingual aspects). These tumours have a marked propensity to spread to the pre-epiglottic space, primarily through fenestrations within the epiglottic cartilage. Moreover they may spread laterally into the hypopharynx or cranially into the oropharynx by extending beyond the aryepiglottic fold.

Glottic tumours arise from the true vocal cords, primarily from the anterior third of the vocal cord. Subglottic tumours are those that involve the true vocal cords with a subglottic extension of more than 1 cm, as well as tumours that are entirely limited to

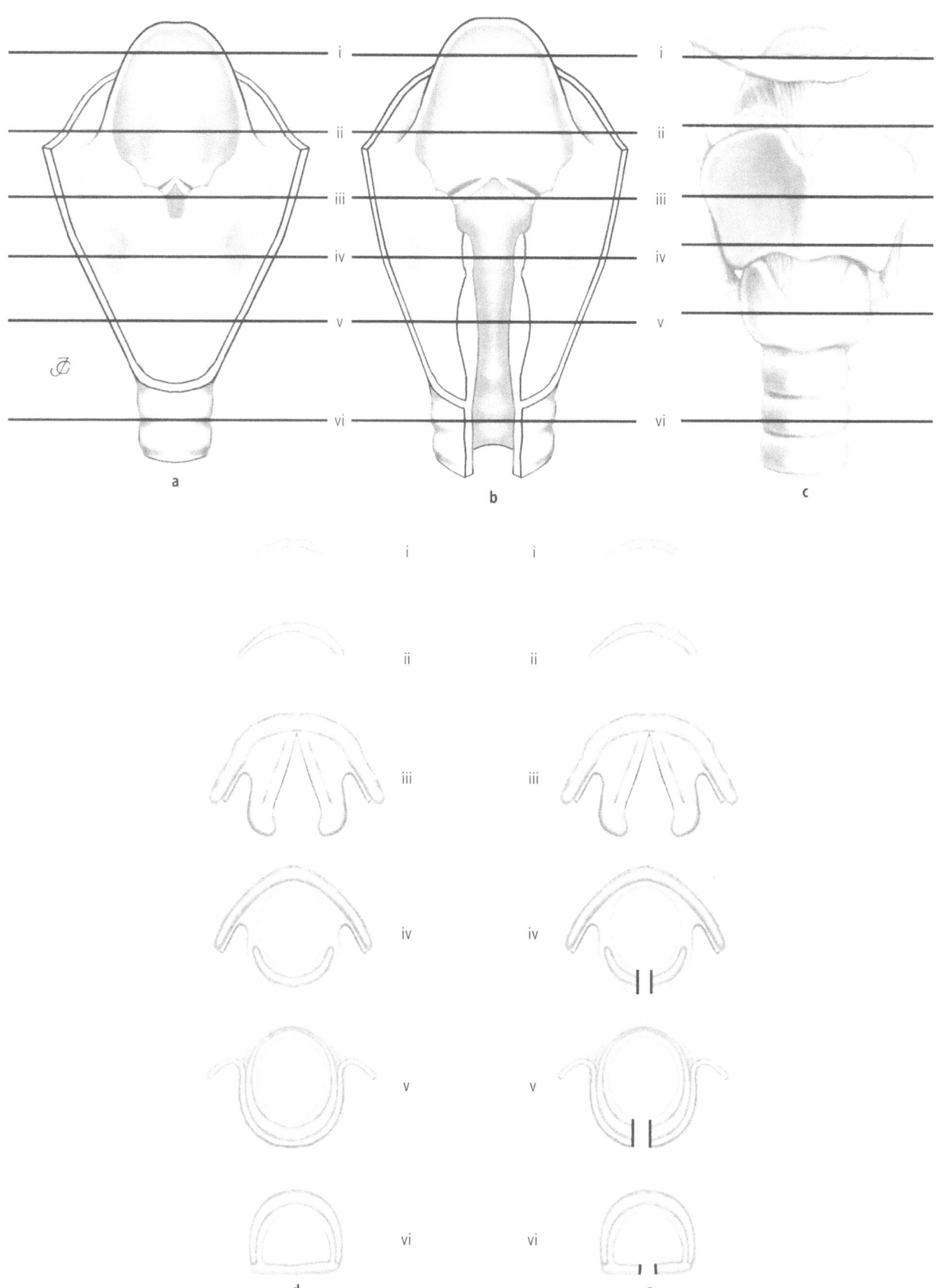

Figure 4.2

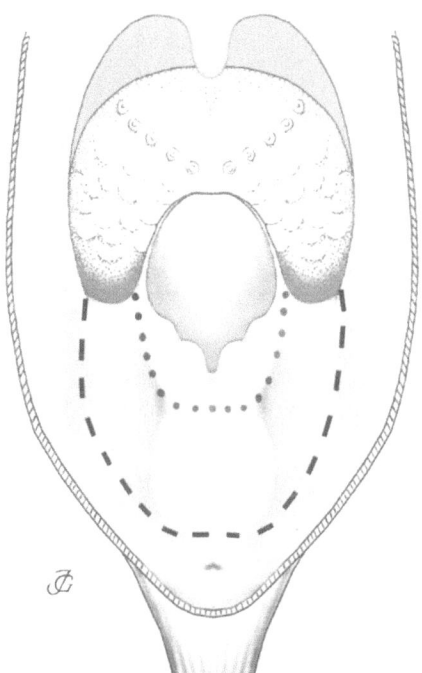

- – – Mucosal extension for hypopharyngeal tumours
- • • • Mucosal extension for endolaryngeal tumours

Larynx and hypopharynx. Posterior view to indicate the extent of hypopharynx that will be removed in the case of hypopharyngeal tumours or endolaryngeal tumours.

Figure 4.3
▲

Pathological anatomy of the larynx.

a Posterior view, larynx closed. Levels of horizontal slices are indicated by lines i–vi.

b Posterior view, larynx opened dorsally. Levels of horizontal slices are indicated by lines i–vi.

c Planes of sectioning projected onto the laryngeal skeleton.

d Horizontal slices from closed larynx. Note that below the level of the tip of the arythenoid cartilages the larynx is a closed tube, more cranial slices (i, ii, iii) being crescents and more caudal slices (iv, v, vi) being closed rings.

e Horizontal slices from a dorsally opened larynx. Slices at levels iv–vi are open dorsally due to opening of the larynx dorsally before slicing.

Figure 4.2
◄

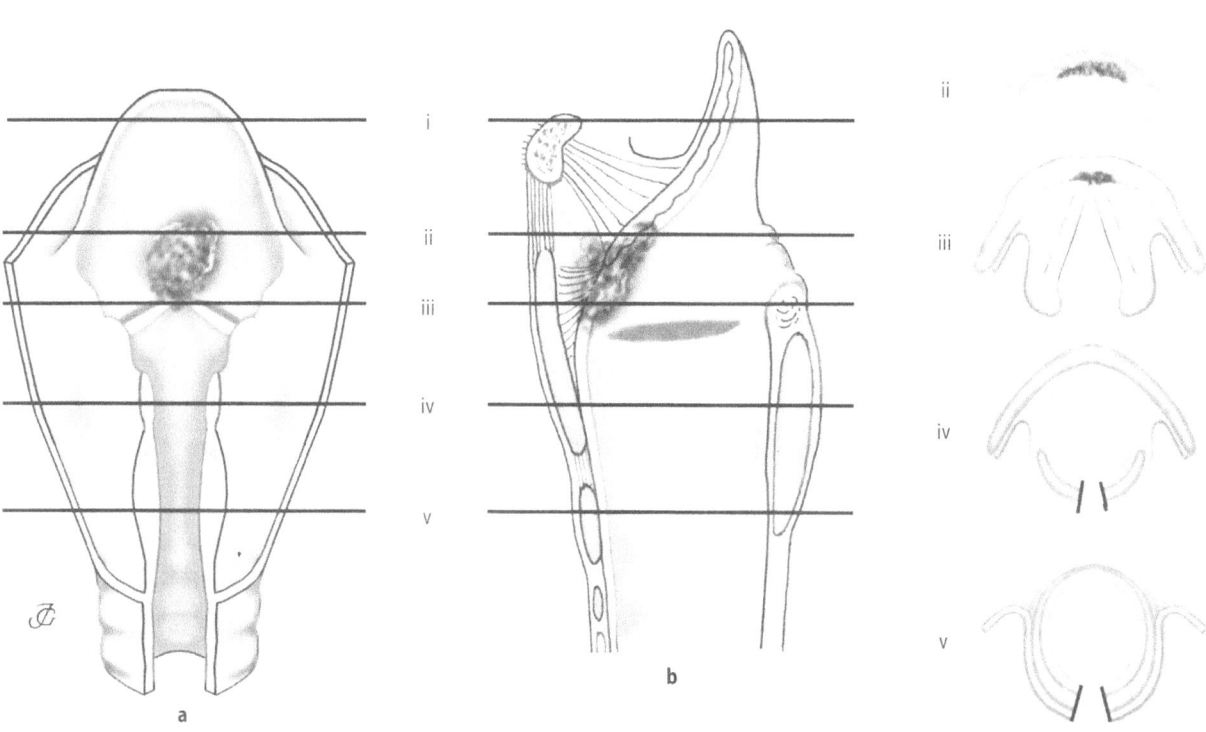

Figure 4.4 Pathological anatomy of supraglottic cancer.

a Clinical appearance when viewed from posterior.

b Sagittal view to display spread into the pre-epiglottic space.

c Slices obtained when cutting the larynx at levels i–v corresponding to the lines shown in **a** and **b**.

the subglottic area. Tumours extending from the supraglottic area into the glottic or even the subglottic region are referred to as transglottic. To make this examination of endolaryngeal tumour extension possible, the larynx has to be opened through a vertical dorsal incision, the line of incision lying just between the two arytenoid cartilages. Usually this incision has already been made by the surgeon.

If the tumour lies in the hypopharynx one should record whether it is located in the pyriform sinus or the postcricoid area. Sometimes both hypopharyngeal areas are involved. Postcricoid cancers may extend into the adjacent cervical oesophagus. Pyriform sinus cancers may extend cranially into the oropharynx or craniomedially into the supraglottic larynx. In the latter case the tumour crosses the aryepiglottic fold that forms the border between hypopharynx and endolarynx.

In resections done for treatment of hypopharyngeal cancers it is better not to open the larynx as this will hamper proper evaluation of the postcricoid area. If the larynx has already been opened on the specimen, one should take the utmost care to discern the caudal mucosal margins that usually are at the border between hypopharynx and oesophagus from margins that are the result of vertical splitting of the larynx and thus do not represent true surgical margins.

Specimens containing the entire larynx and parts of the hypopharynx are cut in horizontal slices. This requires the use of the engine-driven knife as introduced by Michaels and Gregor [2]. The hyoid bone should previously have been removed by sharp dissection from the ventrocranial external laryngeal surface. This bone will be left aside unless histological examination of underlying parts indicates tumour spread into this area; then the hyoid bone has to be histologically investigated also.

Cutting horizontal slices will enable tumour spread, tumour thickness and depth of penetration to be assessed. The tumour spread is dependent on the site of origin. This will be discussed first for endolaryngeal cancers. In the case of supraglottic cancers one has to evaluate whether there is spread anteriorly into the pre-epiglottic space, or growth ventrocranially into the vallecula or base of the tongue (Figs. 4.4, page 70, 4.5, page 72).

Glottic cancers may penetrate the thyroid cartilage when growing laterally or may penetrate into

the extralaryngeal soft tissues through the anterior commissure (Figs. 4.6, page 73, 4.7, page 74). If the tumour penetrates the thyroid cartilage it may involve the medial submucosal tissues of the pyriform sinus. Moreover glottic cancers may grow dorsally between thyroid and arythenoid cartilages and spread into the submucosal tissue of the postcricoid area of the hypopharynx. If this is the case the specimen has two separate caudal surgical margins: the first endolaryngeal and represented by the resection margin through the trachea, the second hypopharyngeal and represented by the resection margin through the postcricoid region.

Subglottic cancers are notorious for their caudal submucosal spread; assessment of this feature, however, requires histological examination in most instances (Figs. 4.8, page 75, 4.9, page 76).

In the case of hypopharyngeal cancers the same horizontal slices as made for evaluation of endolaryngeal cancer will allow assessment of this site. The slices will show the tumour thickness and the depth of penetration. Moreover the minimum distance between tumour front and deep surgical margin can be recorded (Figs. 4.10, page 77, 4.11, page 78). Pyriform sinus cancers may penetrate into this deep surgical margin and extend into the thyroid gland. Medially located cancers may penetrate through the thyroid cartilage to involve the endolaryngeal tissues. In the case of hypopharyngeal cancers located in the postcricoid area or in the caudal part of the pyriform sinus, there may be submucosal spread into the caudal surgical margin that may remain unnoticed if only the mucosal margins of this site are sampled for histological examination; therefore, sections from these margins should also contain adequate submucosal tissue (Figs. 4.12, page 79, 4.13, page 80).

Specific Features

Sometimes tumours are very close to the cranial mucosal margin in the case of lesions situated in the upper part of the pyriform sinus – even extending into the oropharynx – or are close to the ventral mucosal margin in the case of supraglottic lesions that have destroyed the epiglottis. In this case it is better to make the most cranial slice thick, and then to cut it in vertical slices parallel to the long axis of

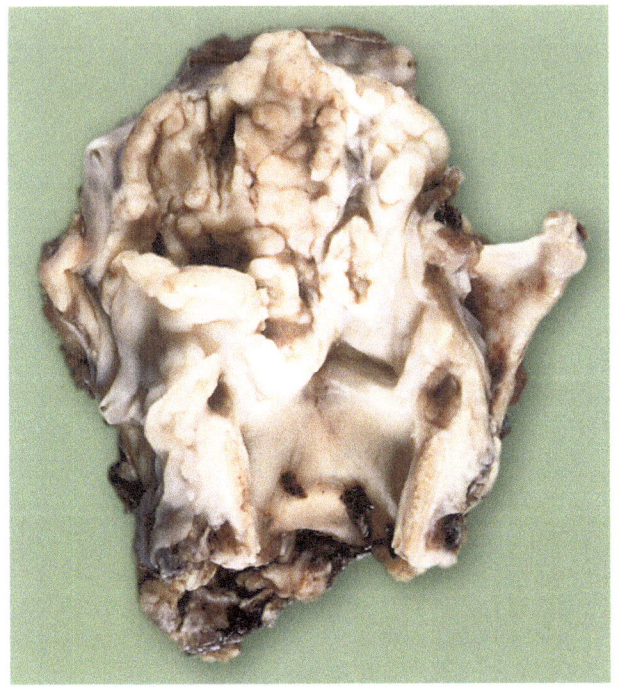

a

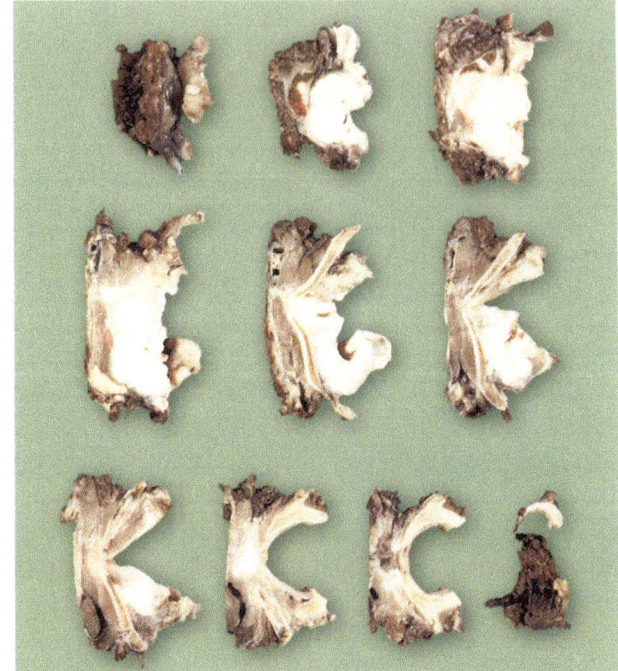

b

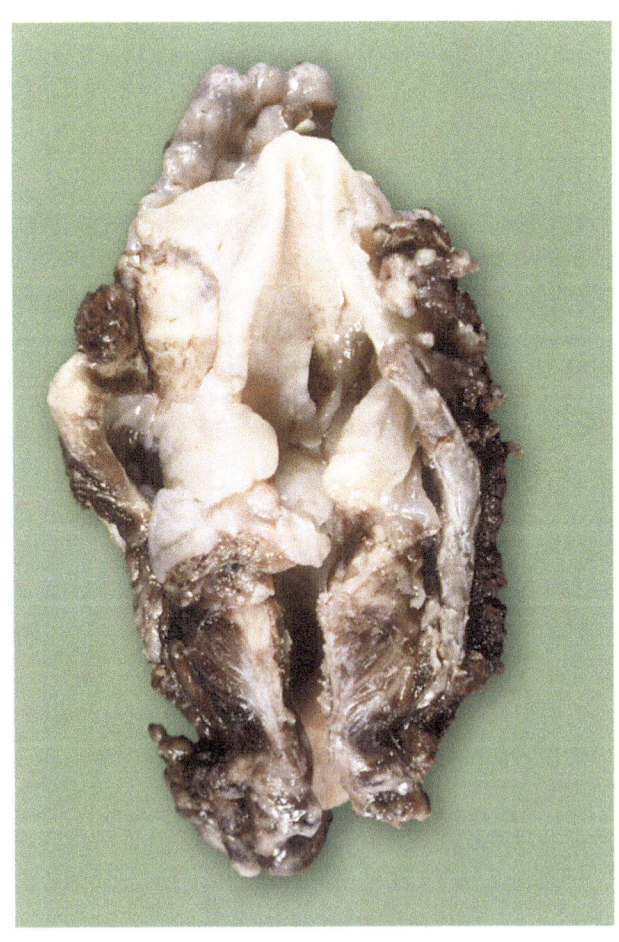

c

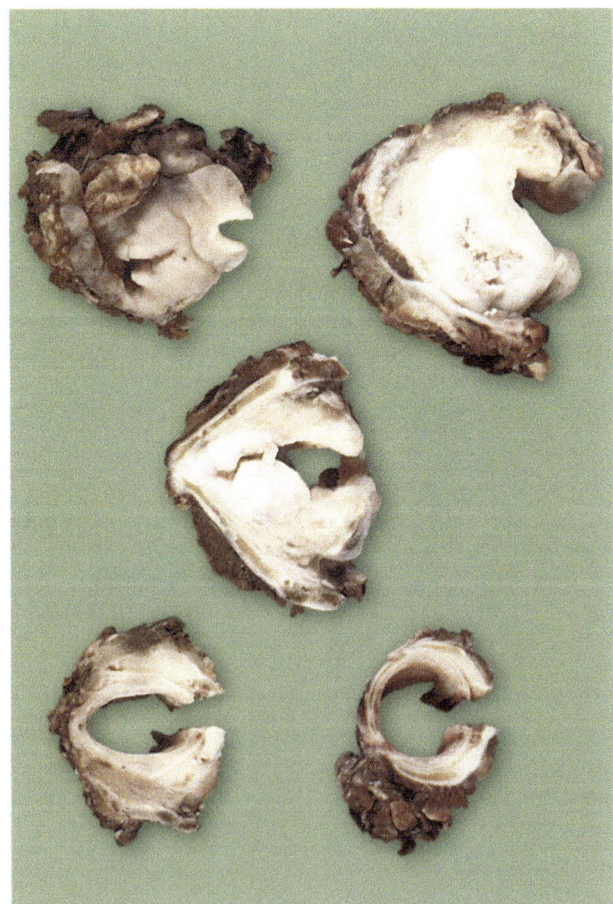

d

Figure 4.5

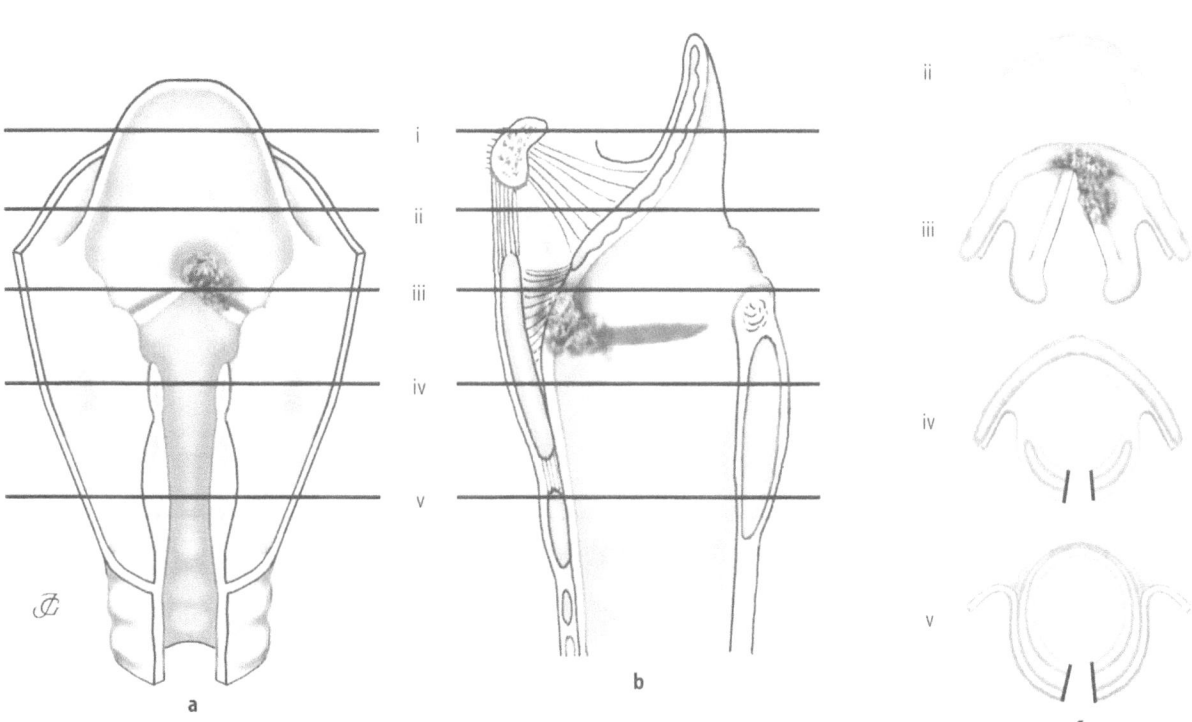

Pathological anatomy of glottic cancer.

a Clinical appearance when viewed from posterior.

b Sagittal view to display involvement of the anterior commissure and spread into the pre-epiglottic space.

c Slices obtained when cutting the larynx at levels i–v corresponding to the lines shown in **a** and **b**.

Figure 4.6
▲

Macroscopic appearances of supraglottic cancers.

a Posterior view of laryngeal specimen showing a huge supraglottic cancer.

b Horizontal slices of the same specimen showing tumour occupying the entire left as well as part of the right supraglottic region.

c Posterior view of a laryngeal specimen in which the supraglottic cancer is characterised by extensive submucosal spread and thus lies underneath a normal mucosal surface. Only the bulging of the mucosa indicates the presence of tumour. This supraglottic tumour manifestation may be confused with cancer of the vallecula.

d Horizontal slices of the same specimen showing extensive tumour spread in the supraglottic region.

Figure 4.5
◄

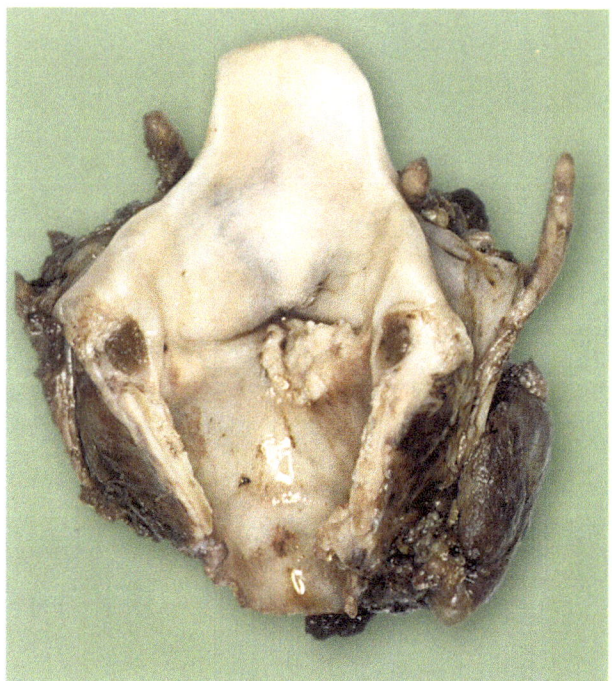

a

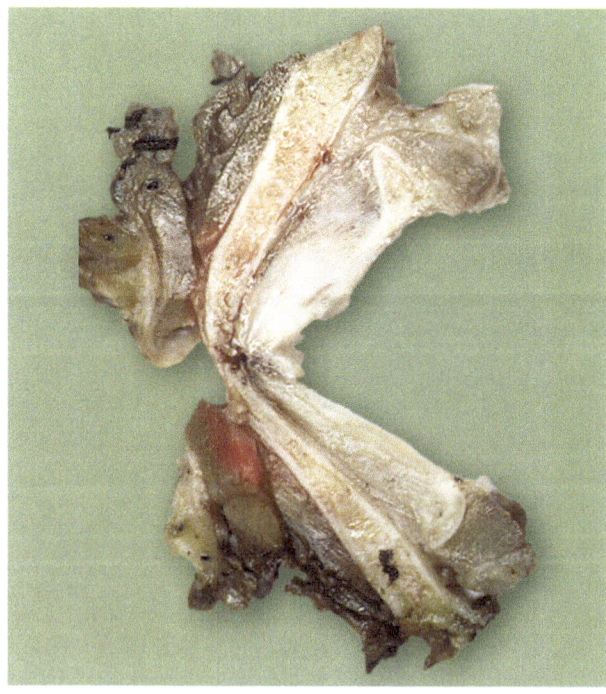

b

Figure 4.7 Macroscopic appearance of glottic cancer.

a Posterior view showing tumour at the right vocal fold.

b Horizontal slice at the glottic level showing tumour confined to the right half of the larynx and not penetrating into the adjacent thyroid cartilage.

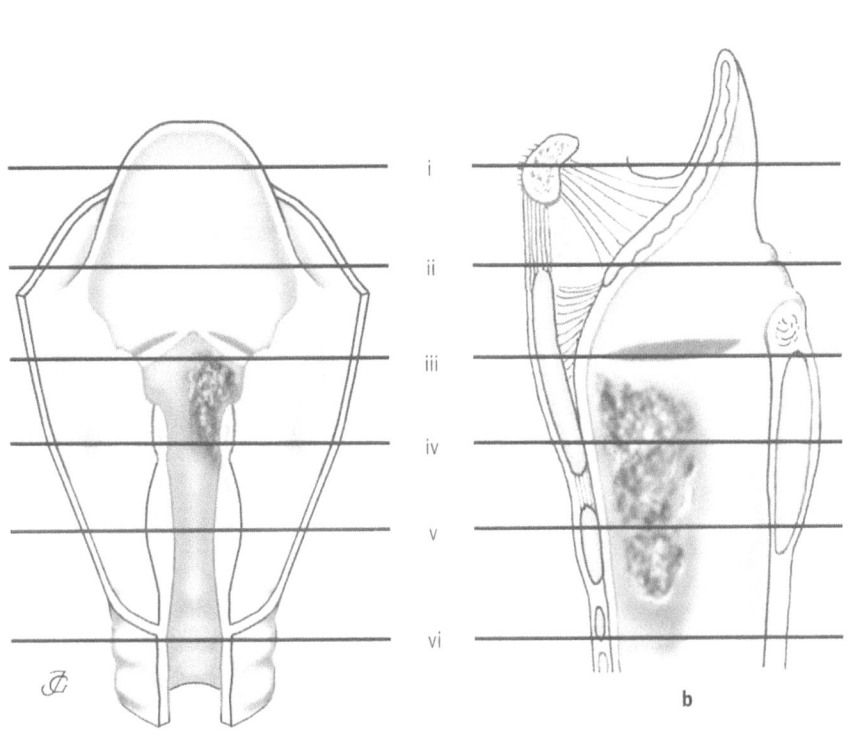

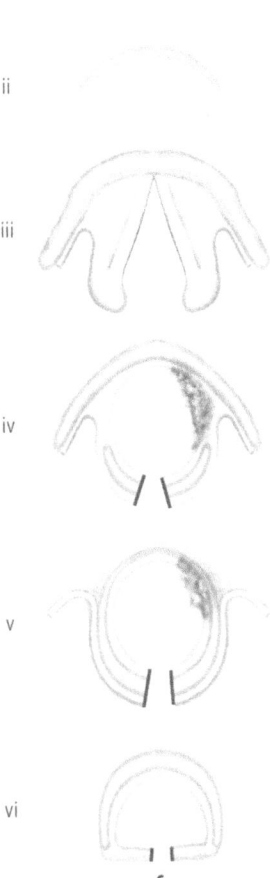

Pathological anatomy of subglottic cancer.

a Clinical appearance when viewed from posterior.

b Sagittal view to display tumour extension.

c Slices obtained when cutting the larynx at levels i–vi corresponding to the lines shown in **a** and **b**.

Figure 4.8
▲

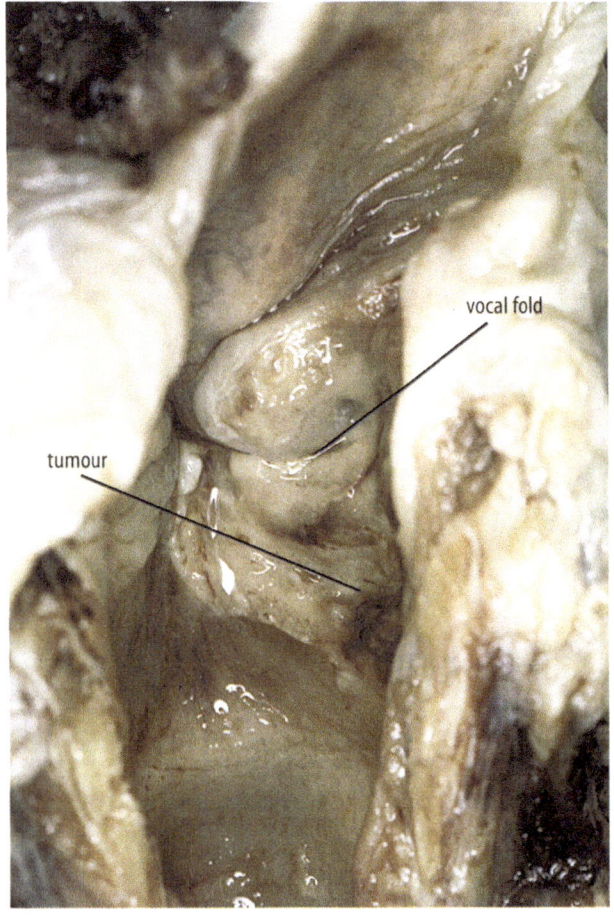

a

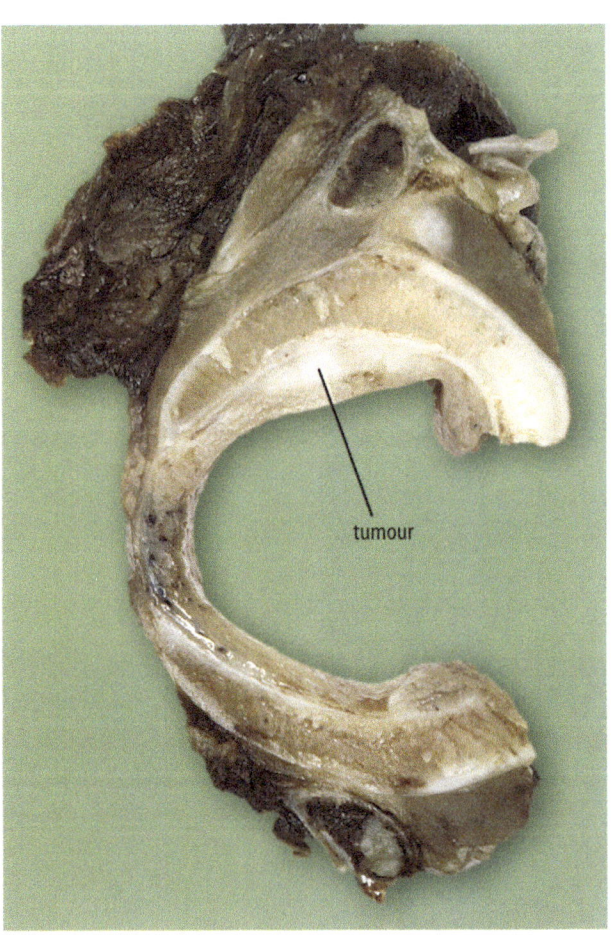

b

Figure 4.9
▲

a Macroscopic appearance of subglottic cancer.

b Horizontal slice showing submucosal caudal tumour extension.

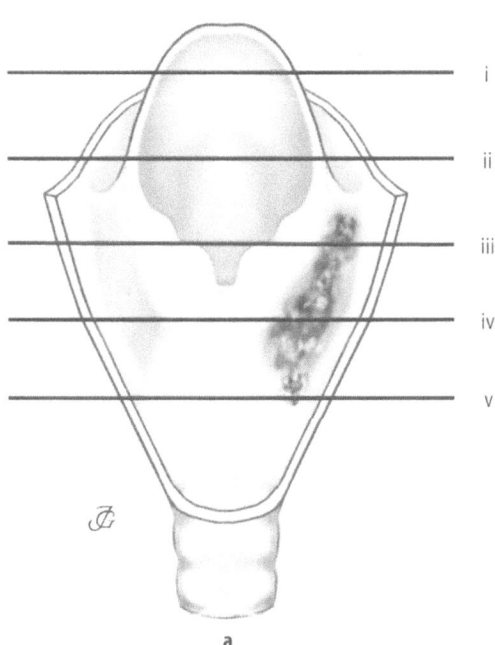

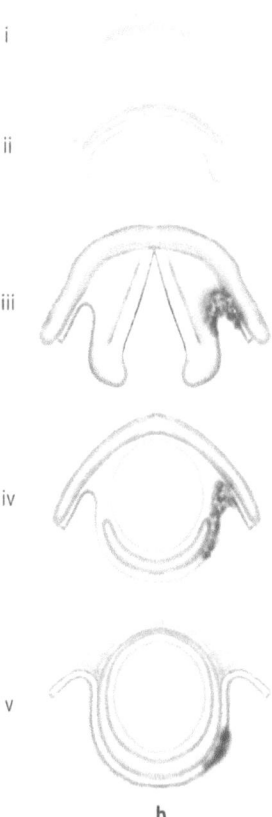

Pathological anatomy of pyriform sinus cancer.

a Clinical appearance when viewed from posterior.

b Slices obtained when cutting the larynx at levels i–v corresponding to the lines shown in **a**.

Figure 4.10
▲

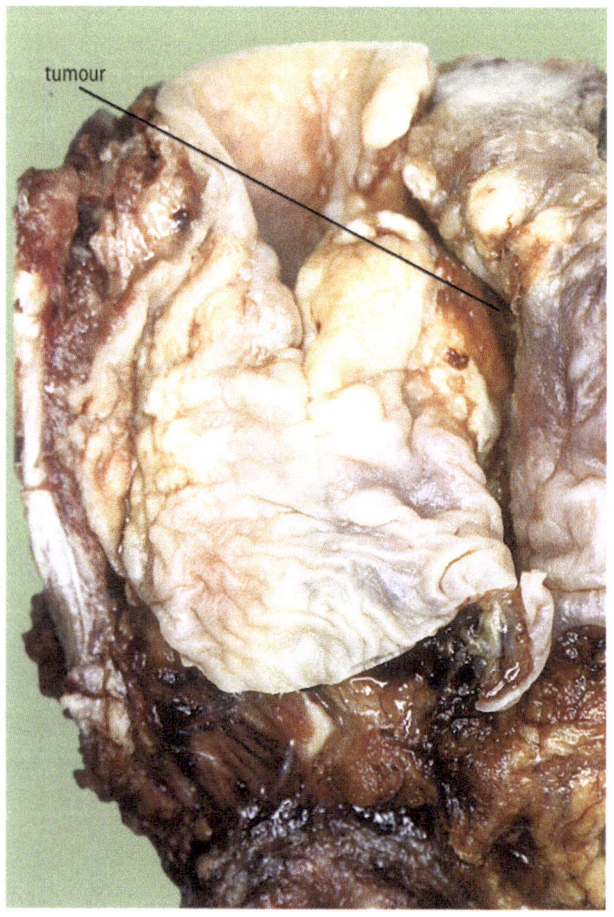

a

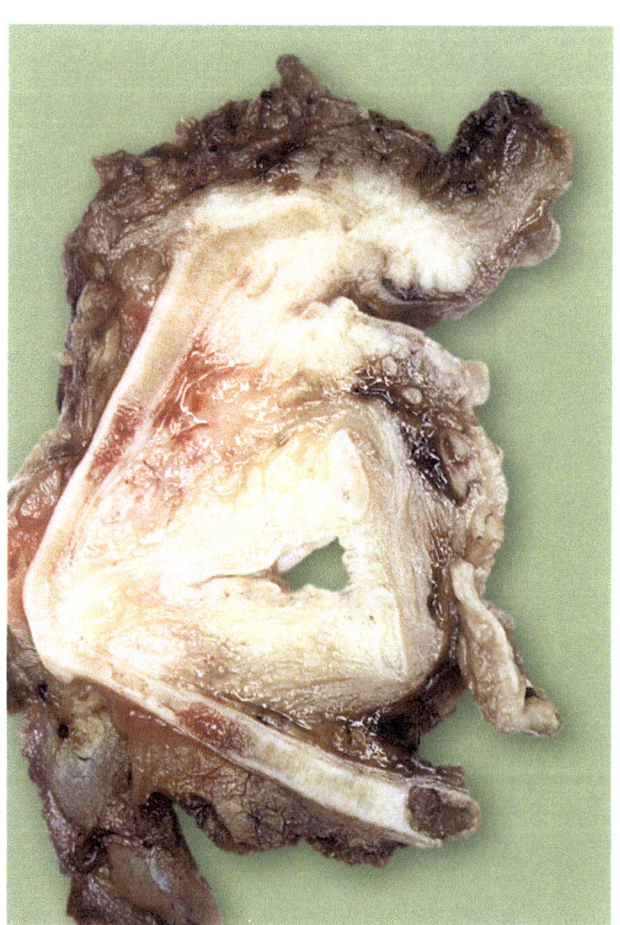

b

Figure 4.11
▲

a Macroscopic appearance of cancer in the right pyriform sinus.

b Horizontal slice showing tumour in the pyriform sinus extending medially as well as laterally and laterally borderered by the thyroid cartilage.

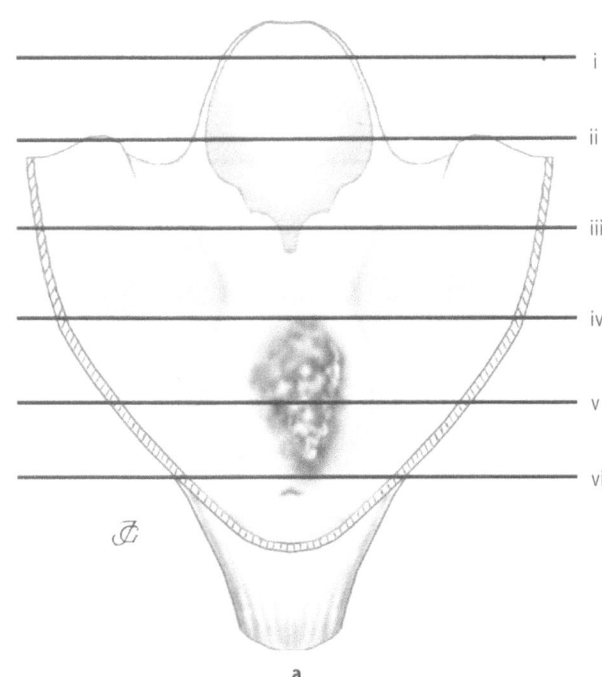

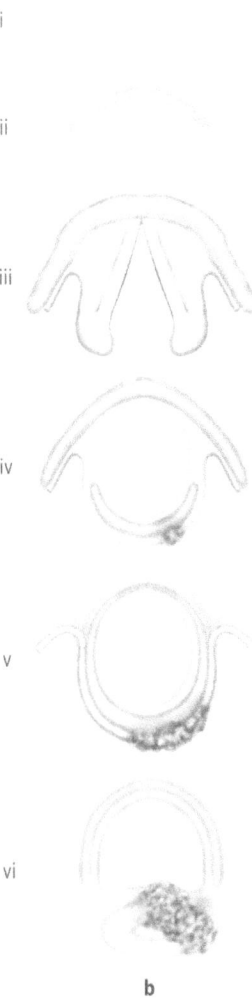

Pathological anatomy of postcricoid cancer.

a Clinical appearance when viewed from posterior.

b Slices obtained when cutting the larynx at levels i–vi corresponding to the lines shown in **a**. At level vi tumour extends into the oesophageal entrance.

Figure 4.12
▲

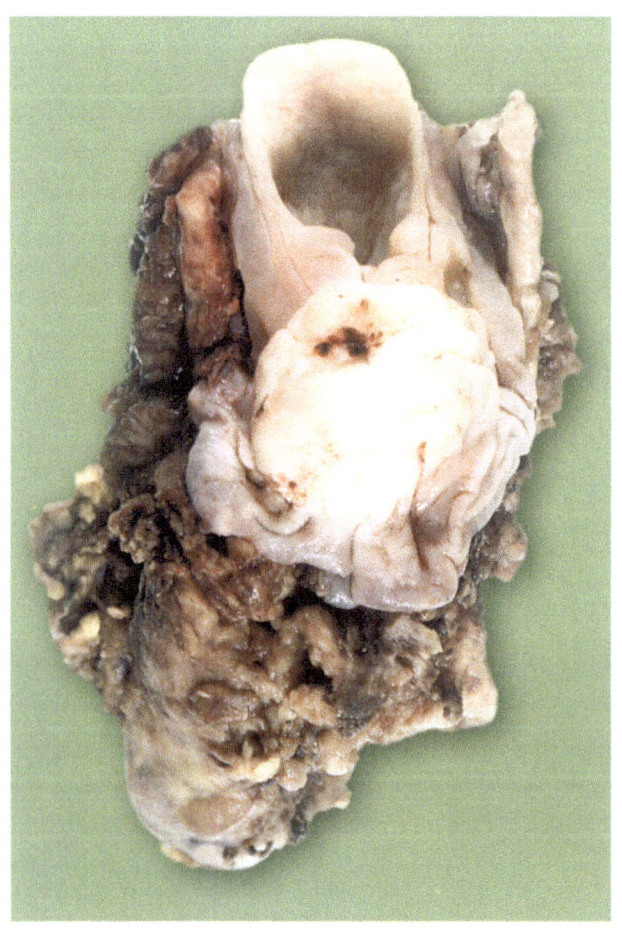

a

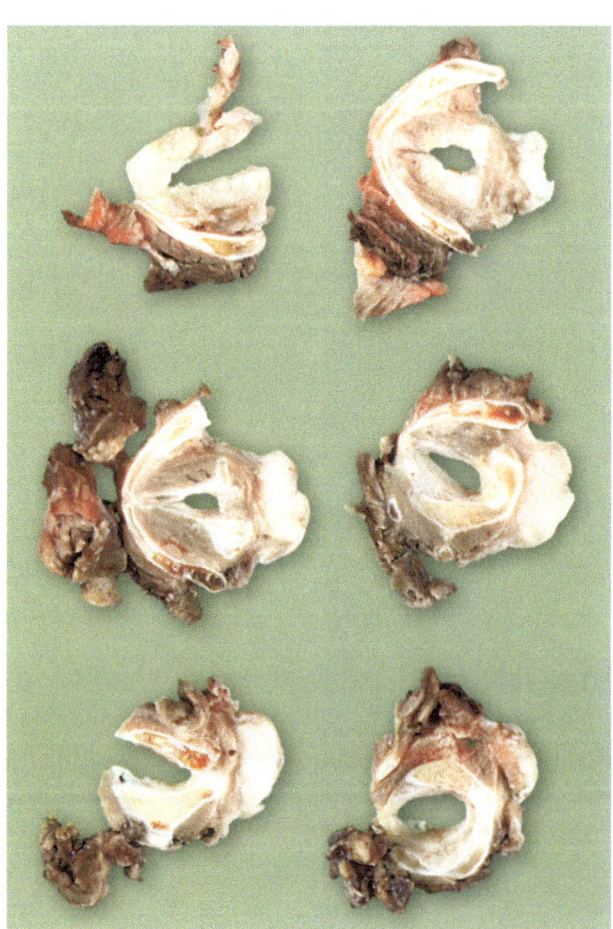

b

Figure 4.13
a Macroscopic appearance of postcricoid cancer located between the laryngeal and oesophageal entrance.

b Horizontal slices showing tumour located dorsal to the arythenoid cartilages.

the larynx. In this way it is easier to examine the minimum distance between invading tumour front and deep muscular as well as superficial mucosal margin in this part of the specimen. Similarly, it is better to cut vertical slices from the caudal part of the specimen if tumours in the pyriform sinus or postcricoid area lie very close to the caudal margin (Figs. 4.14–4.23, pages 82–91).

In the case of a horizontal hemilaryngectomy this supraglottic part of the larynx can be handled in the same way as outlined for specimens containing whole laryngectomies (Figs. 4.24, page 92, 4.25, page 93). In the case of a vertical hemilaryngectomy the rectangular specimen is unilaterally covered with a mucosal surface that shows a longitudinal cleft representing the entrance to the ventricle, the vocal cord representing the lower border of this cleft. These specimens are cut in parallel slices perpendicular to the vocal cord. Slices thus obtained show the supraglottic area of the false vocal cords, the ventricle and the vocal cord, and the cranial part of the subglottic area (Fig. 4.26, page 93).

If the laryngectomy specimen contains a tracheostoma, the relationship between stoma and tumour should be recorded. Moreover the margins through the skin surface of the stoma should be sampled for histological examination (Fig. 4.27, page 94).

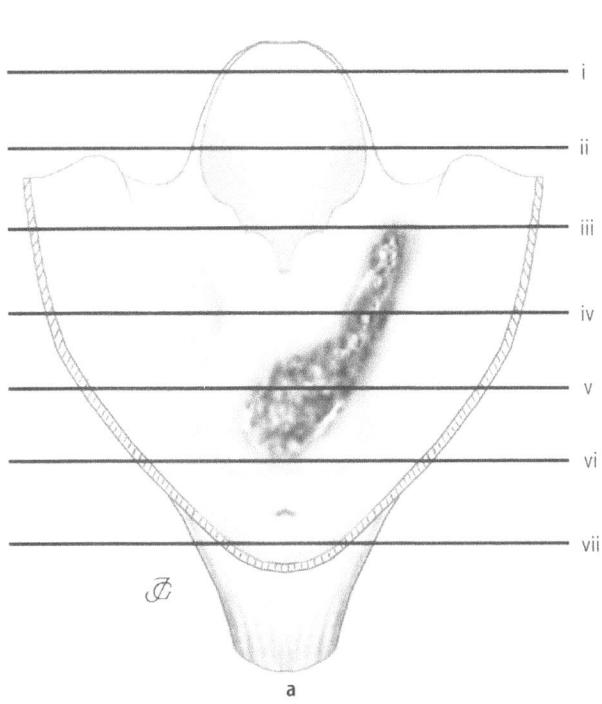

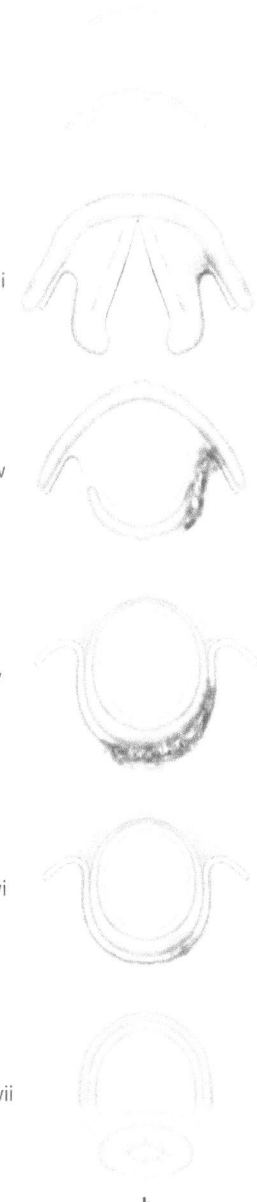

Figure 4.14 Pathological anatomy of pyriform sinus cancer spreading into the postcricoid region.

a Clinical appearance when viewed from posterior.

b Slices obtained when cutting the larynx at levels i–vii corresponding to the lines shown in **a**.

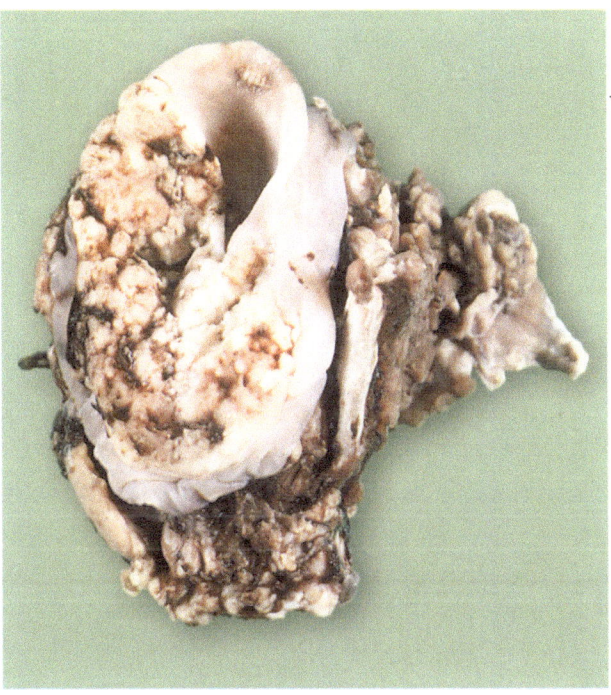

a

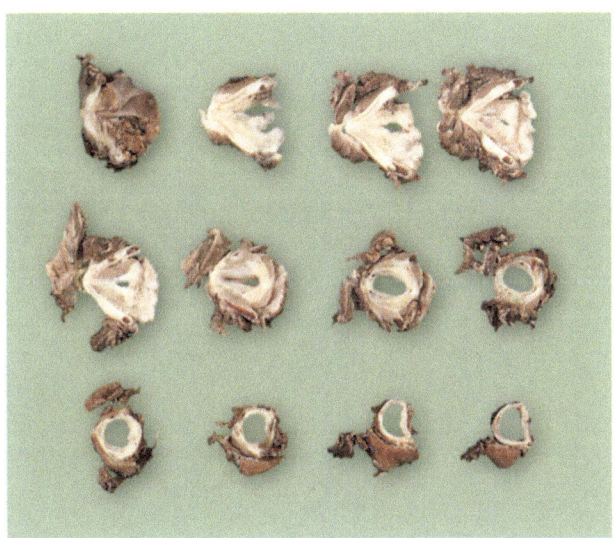

b

a Macroscopic appearance of cancer in the left pyriform sinus extending mediocaudally into the postcricoid area.

b Horizontal slices visualising tumour size and extension.

Figure 4.15
▲

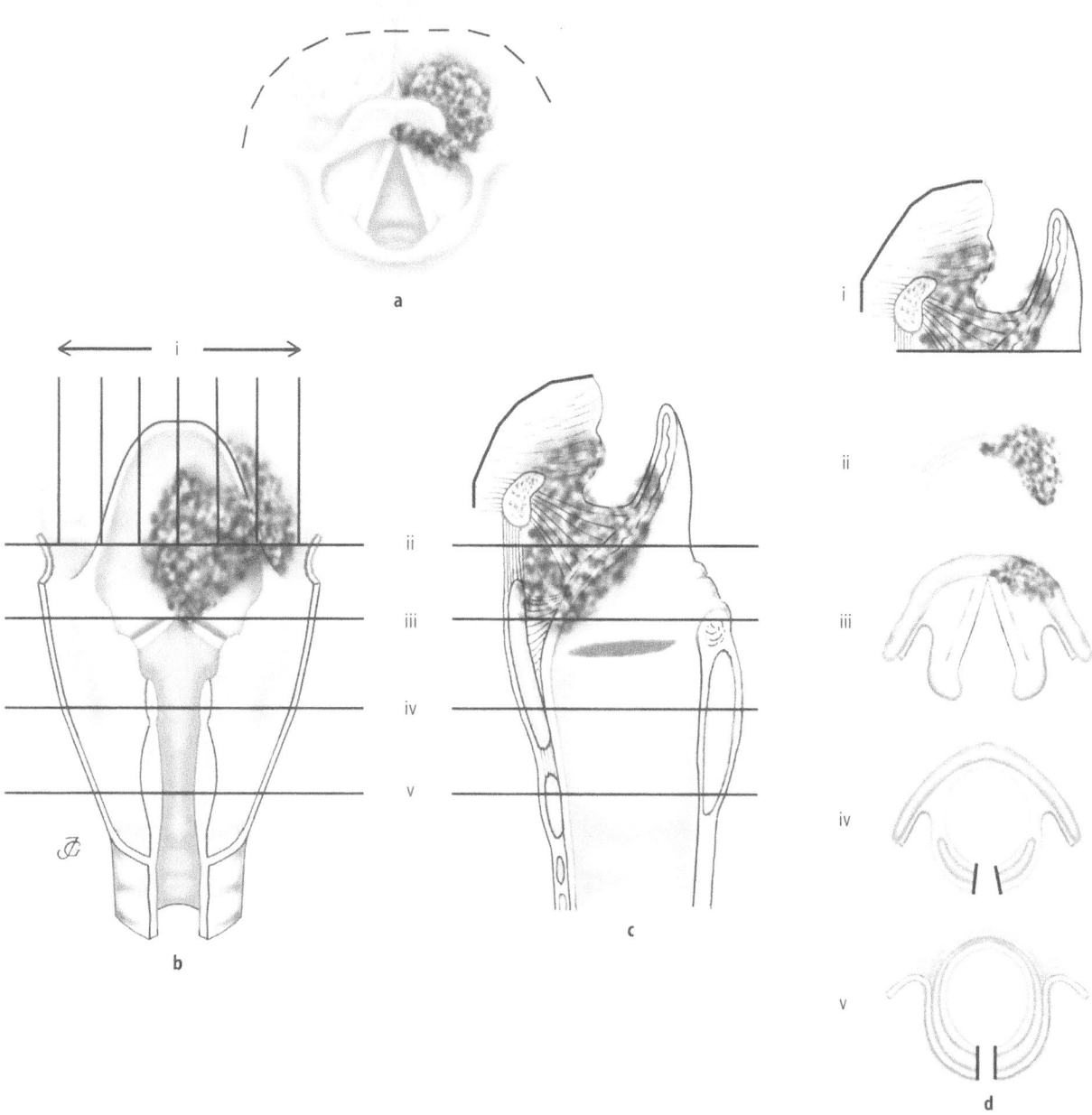

Figure 4.16
▲

Pathological anatomy of supraglottic endolaryngeal cancer spreading into the hypopharynx laterally and oropharynx cranially.

a Clinical *appearance as shown by laryngoscopy. Dashed line indicates* the ventral outline of the resection.

b Appearance of surgical specimen when viewed from posterior.

c Sagittal view to show tumour extension into the base of the tongue ventrally. A line is drawn through the base of the tongue to indicate the ventral outline of the resection.

d Slices obtained when cutting the larynx at levels i–v corresponding to the lines shown in **b** and **c**. Note that the upper half of the supraglottic region is sliced sagittally as indicated by line i; the remainder of the specimen is sliced horizontally as indicated by lines ii–v.

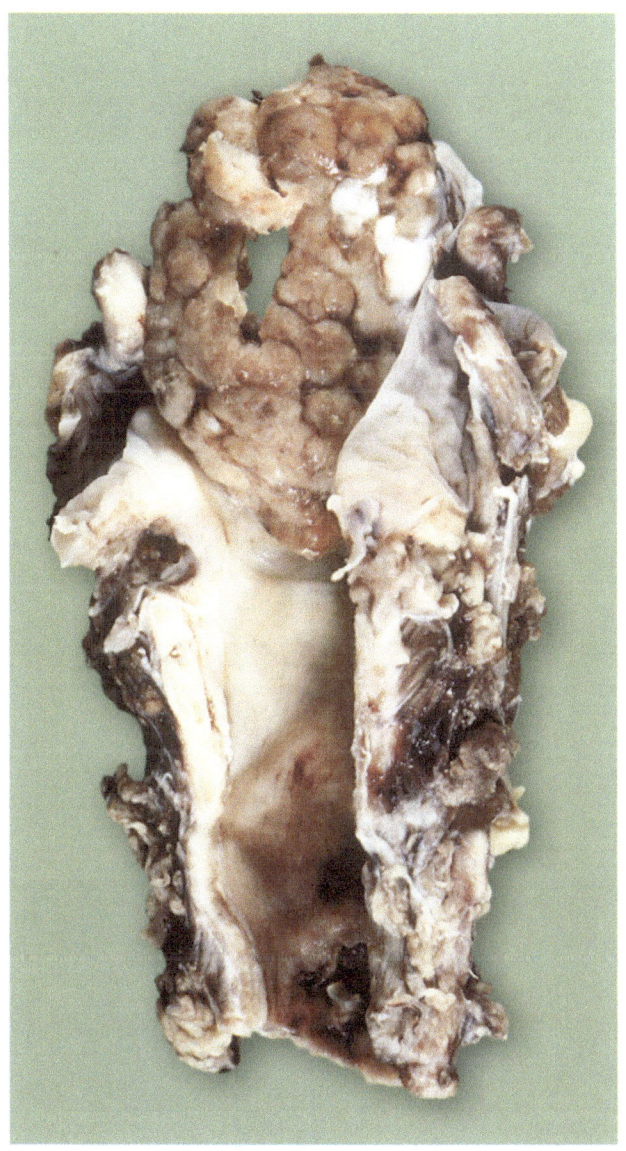

a

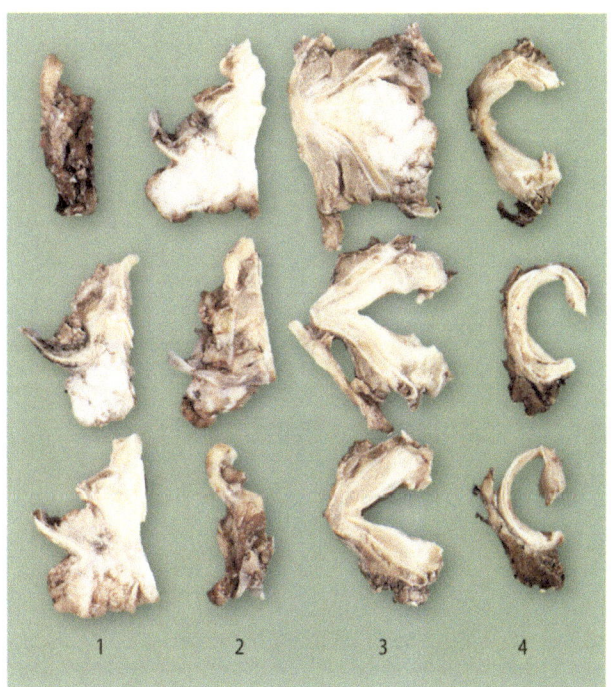

1   2   3   4

b

a Macroscopic appearance of cancer involving both the supraglottic and oropharyngeal regions.

b Slices allowing evaluation of tumour size and extension. Vertical rows 1 and 2 show slices made sagittally whereas vertical rows 3 and 4 show slices made horizontally as outlined in Fig. 4.16.

Figure 4.17
▲

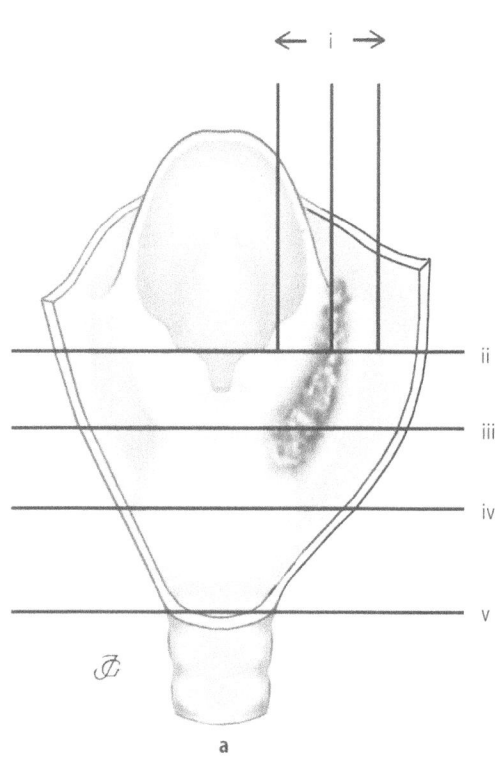

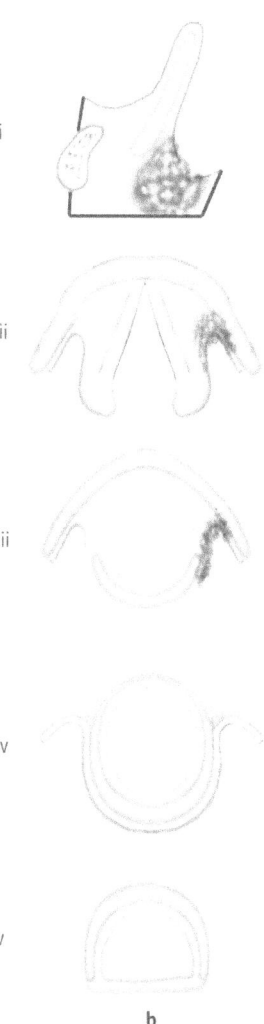

Figure 4.18   Pathological anatomy of pyriform sinus cancer spreading into the oropharynx cranially.

a Clinical appearance when viewed from posterior.

b Slices obtained when cutting the larynx at levels i–v corresponding to the lines shown in **a**.
Note that the cranial part of the hypopharyngeal region is sliced sagittally as indicated by
line i. The remainder of the specimen is sliced horizontally as indicated by lines ii–v.

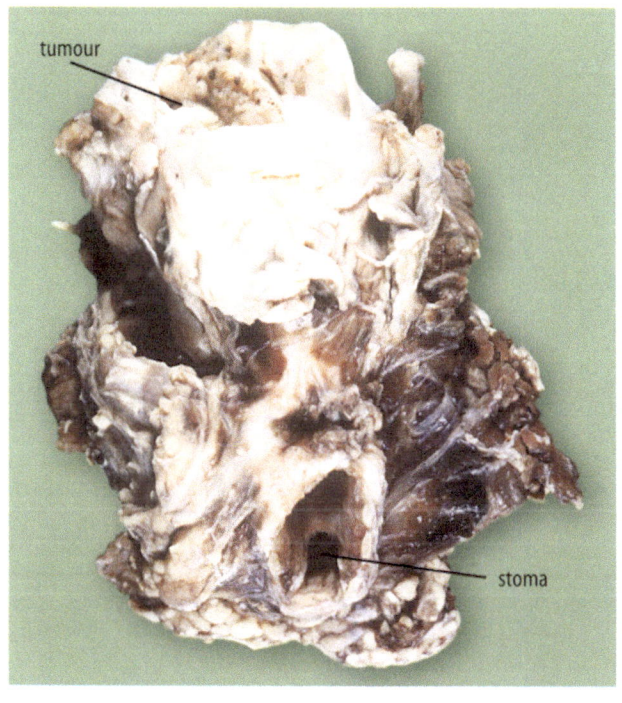

tumour

stoma

a

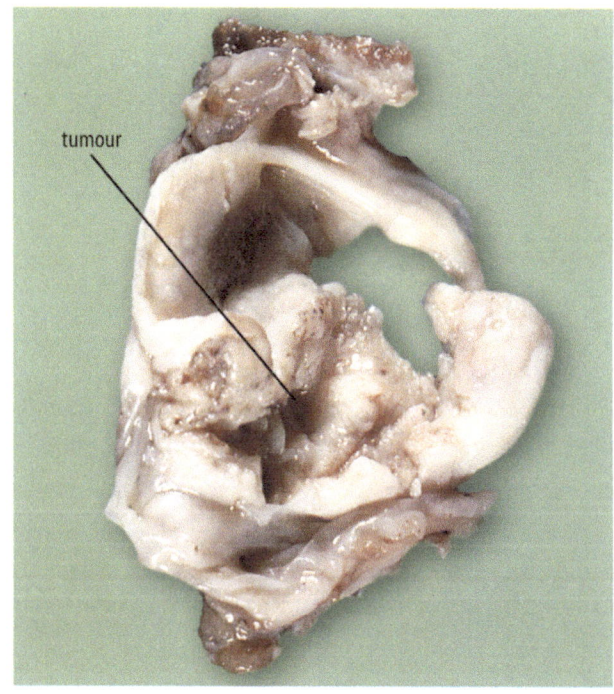

tumour

b

c

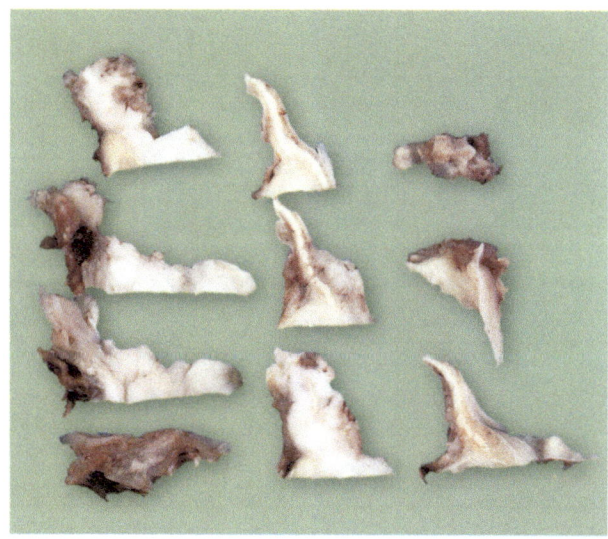

d

a Macroscopic appearance of cancer in the cranial part of the pyriform sinus extending into the oropharynx cranially. Tracheal stoma is shown also.

b Cranial view showing tumour involving the lateral part of the epiglottis, dorsal part of the vallecula and cranial part of the pyriform sinus.

c Specimen sliced horizontally to display tumour spread into the supraglottic and pyriform sinus areas.

d Cranial part of the specimen sliced sagittally showing tumour spread anteriorly and cranially.

Figure 4.19
▲

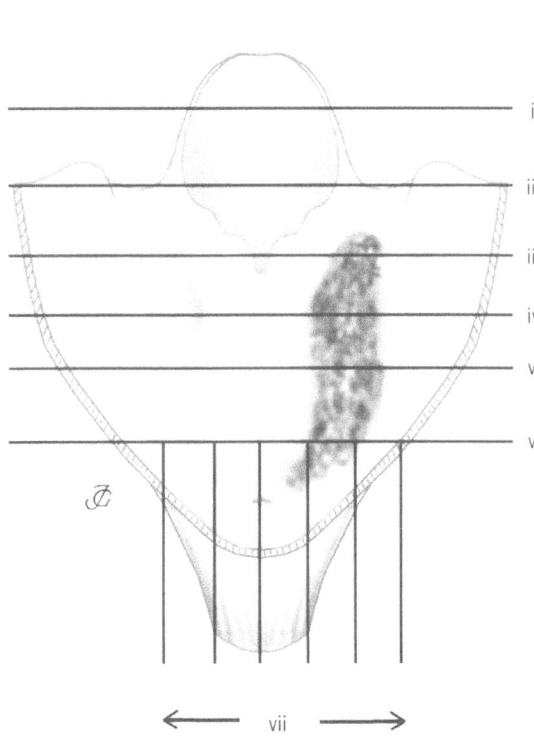

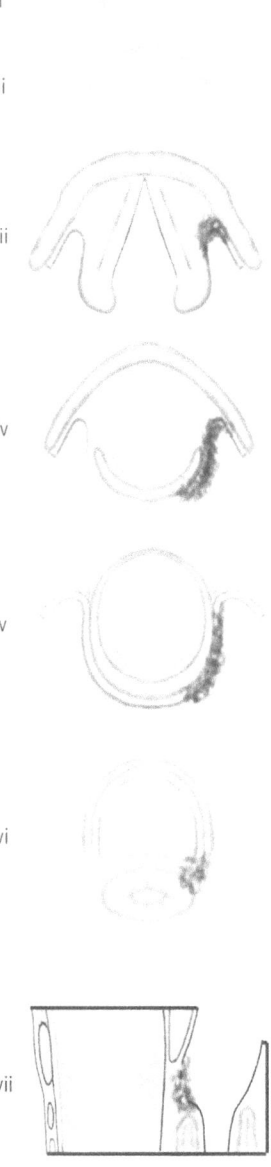

a

b

Figure 4.20
▲

Pathological anatomy of pyriform sinus cancer lying close to the junction of the hypopharynx with the oesophagus.

a Clinical appearance when viewed from posterior.

b Slices obtained when cutting the larynx at levels i–vii corresponding to the lines shown in **a**. Note that the caudal part of the hypopharyngeal region is sliced sagittally as indicated by line vii; the remainder of the specimen is sliced horizontally as indicated by lines i–vi.

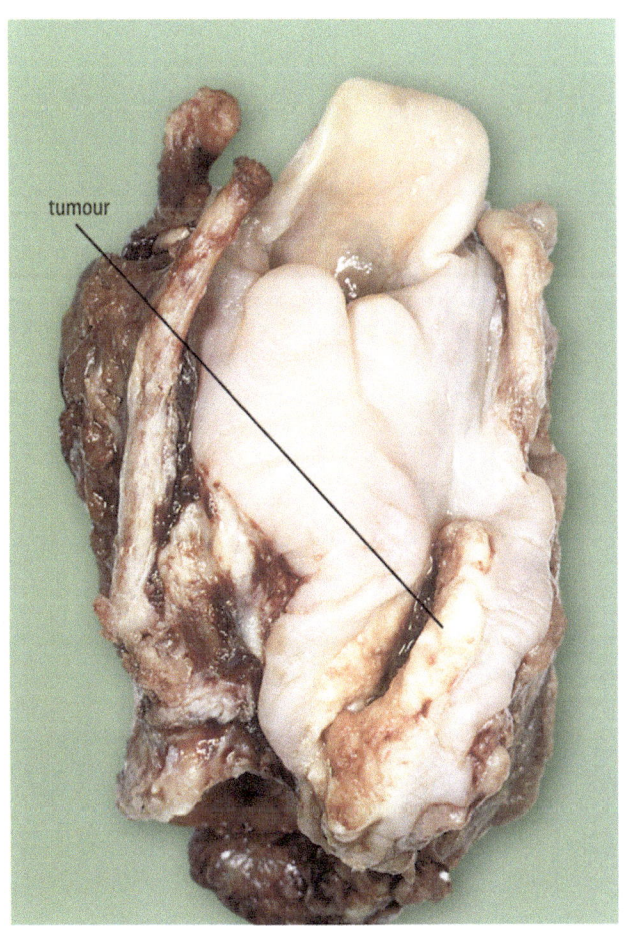

a

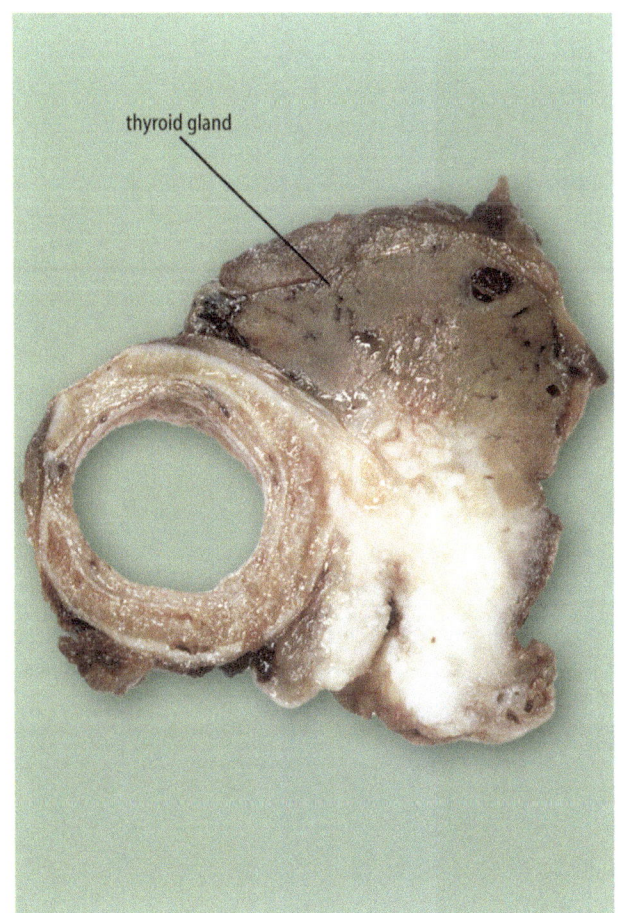

b

a Macroscopic appearance of caudally located pyriform sinus cancer.

b Horizontal slice showing tumour spread into the adjacent thyroid gland.

Figure 4.21
▲

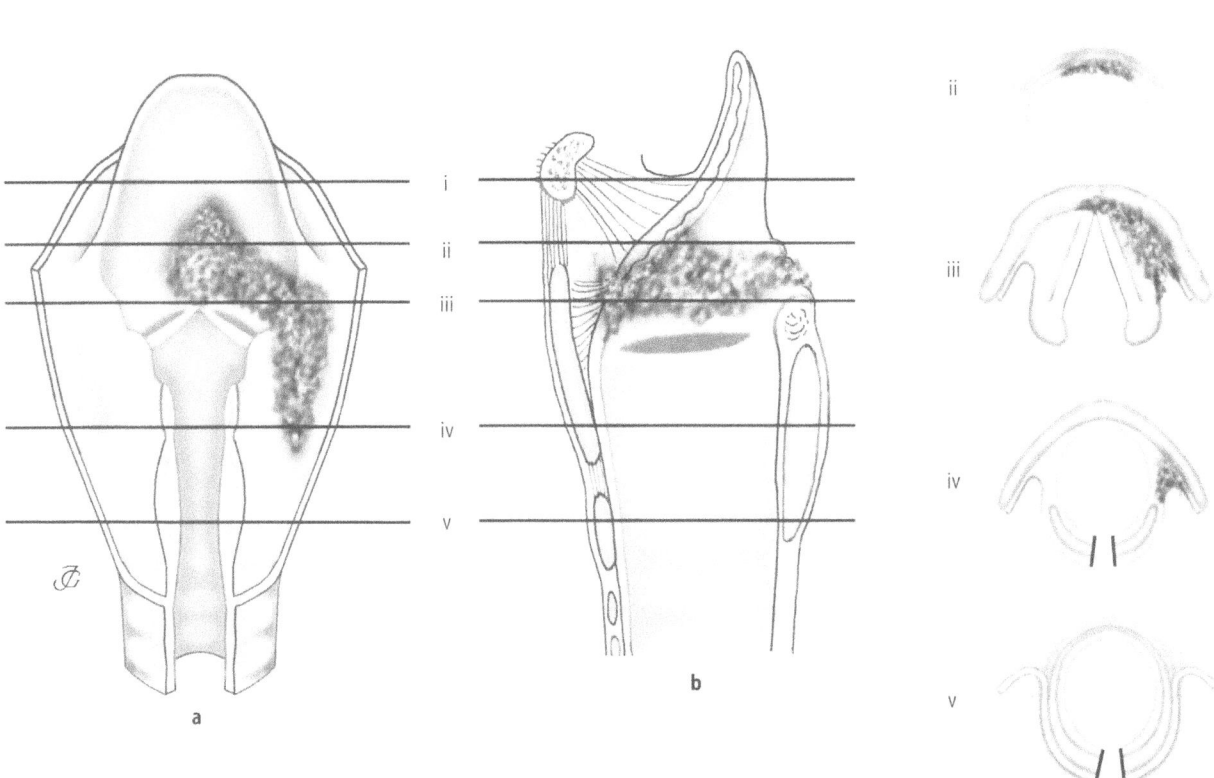

Figure 4.22
▲

Pathological anatomy of supraglottic cancer extending laterally into the pyriform sinus.

a Clinical appearance when viewed from posterior.

b Sagittal view to display involvement of the epiglottis and spread into the pre-epiglottic space.

c Slices obtained when cutting the larynx at levels i–v corresponding to the lines shown in **a** and **b**.

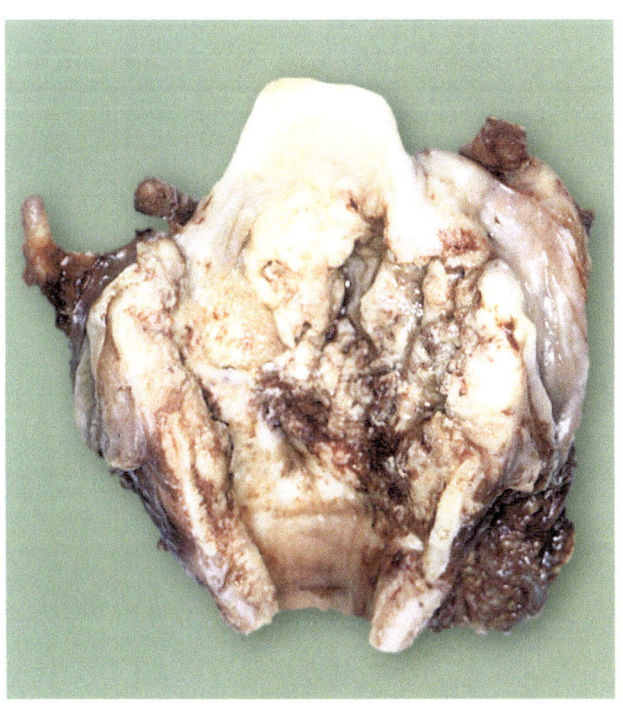

a

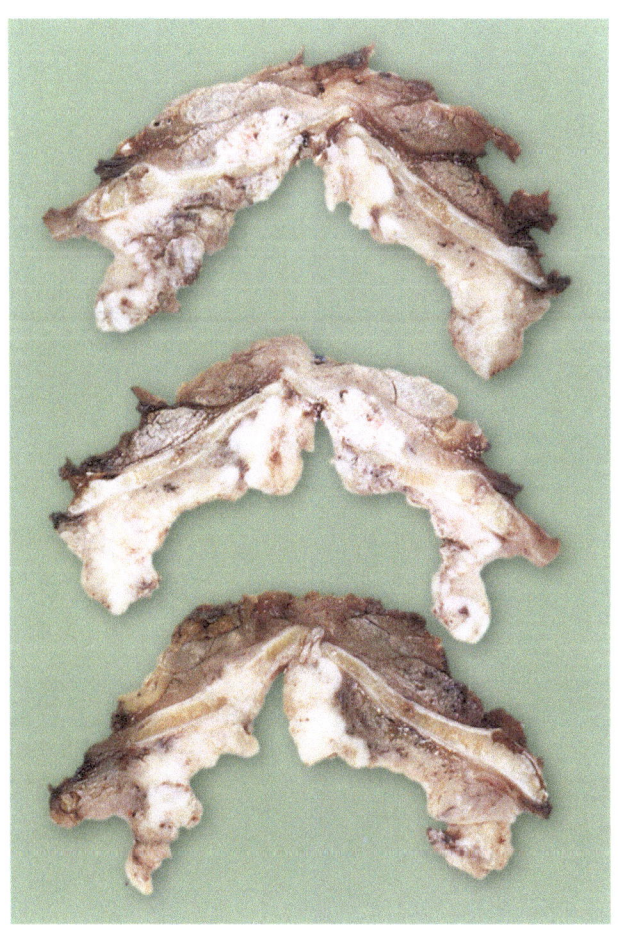

b

a Macroscopic appearance of glottic–supraglottic cancer extending laterally into the adjacent pyriform sinus.

b Horizontal slices showing tumour located endolaryngeally as well as in the pyriform sinus. Destruction of the thyroid cartilage is also present.

Figure 4.23
▲

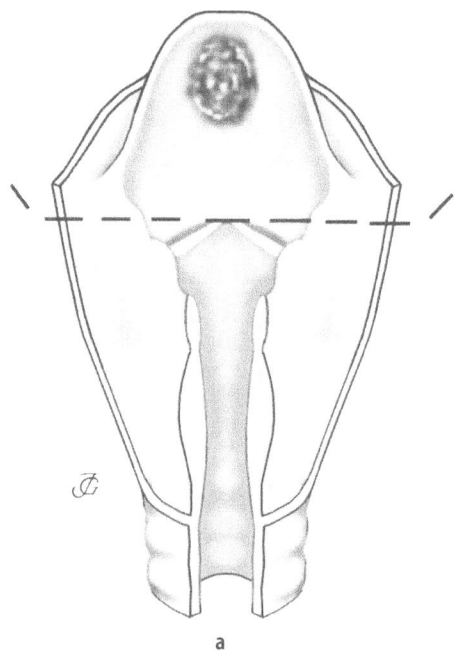

a

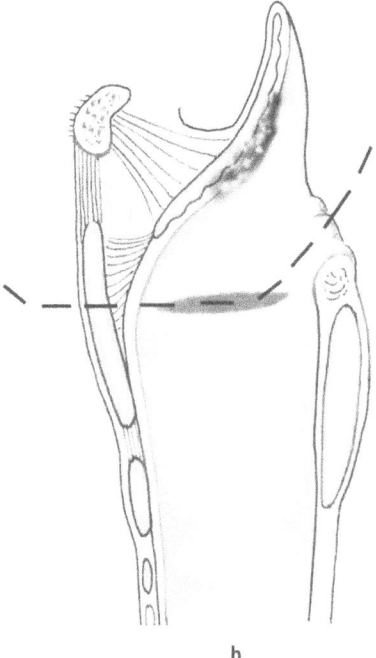

b

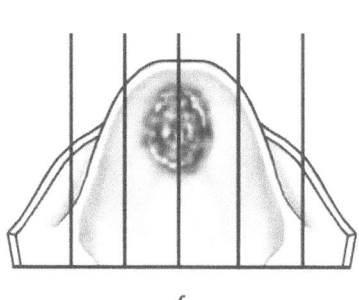

c

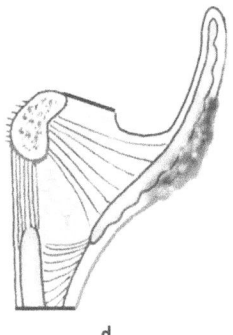

d

Figure 4.24
▲

Pathological anatomy of small supraglottic cancers allowing horizontal hemilaryngectomy.

a Clinical appearance when viewed from posterior.

b Sagittal view to display involvement of the epiglottis and outline of the resection.

c Surgical specimen and plane of sectioning.

d Cut surface displaying tumour site and size.

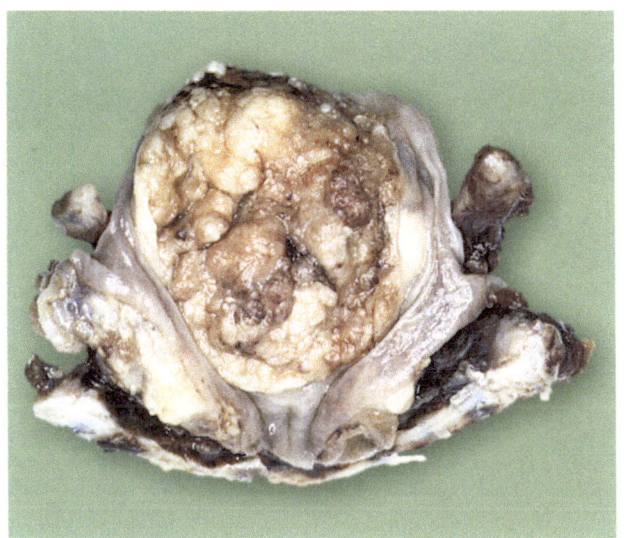

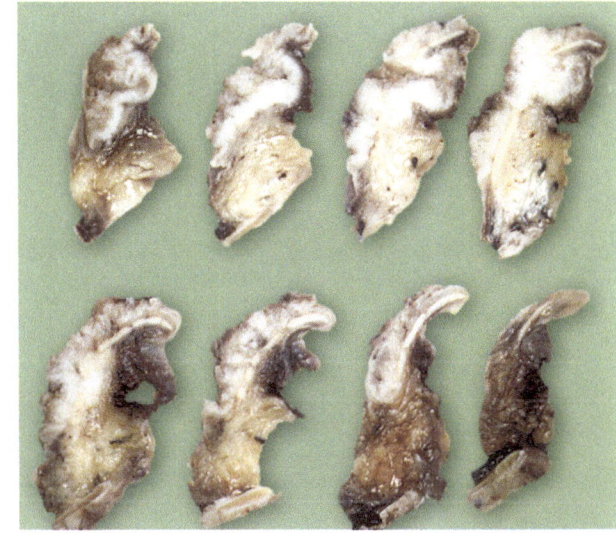

a

b

a Macroscopic appearance of specimen obtained by horizontal hemilaryngectomy. Tumour is present at the laryngeal side of the epiglottis.

b Sagittal slices showing tumour present on both sides of the epiglottis.

Figure 4.25
▲

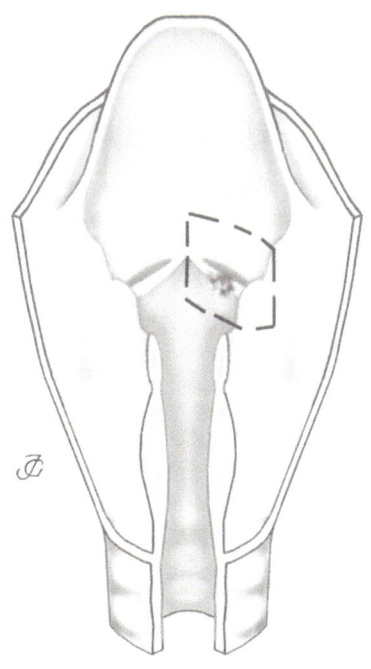

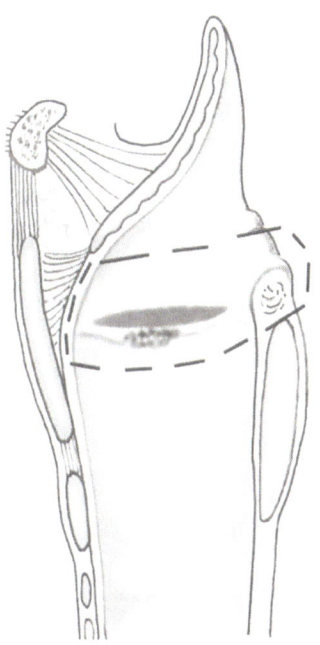

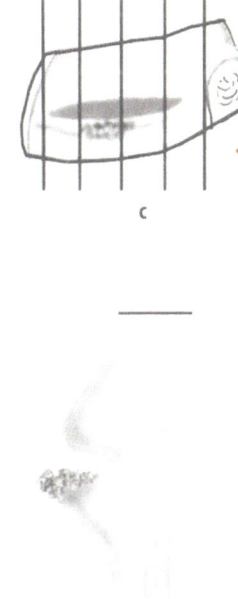

c

a

b

d

Pathological anatomy of small unilateral glottic cancers allowing vertical hemilaryngectomy.

a Clinical appearance when viewed from posterior.

b Sagittal view to display involvement of the glottis and outline of the resection.

c Surgical specimen and plane of sectioning.

d Cut surface displaying tumour site and size.

Figure 4.26
▲

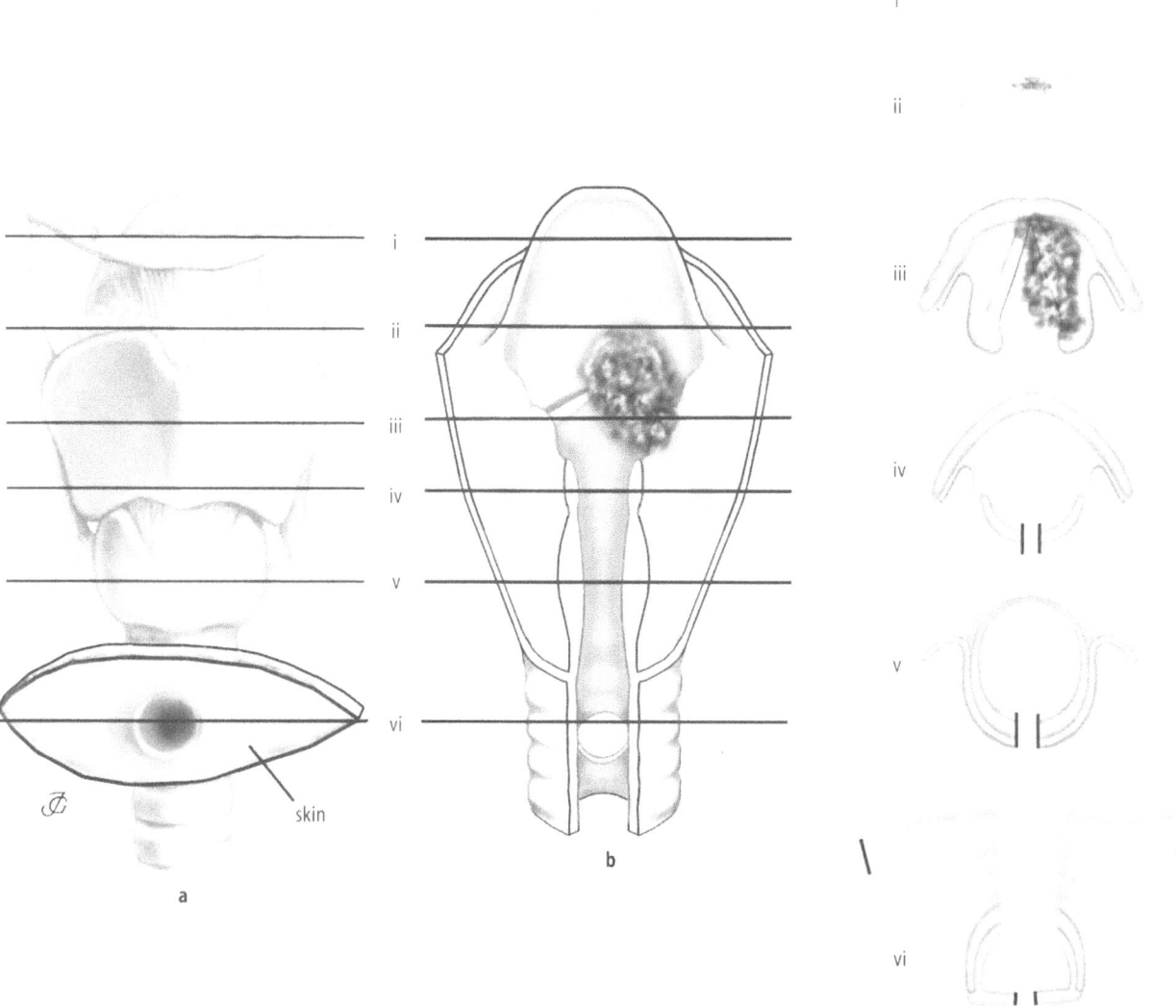

Figure 4.27 Pathological anatomy of endolaryngeal cancer with tracheostoma.

a Anterior view to show location of the stoma.

b Posterior view to show endolaryngeal cancer and tracheal side of the stoma. Lines i–vi indicate planes of sectioning.

c Horizontal slices obtained when cutting horizontally at levels i–vi. Slice vi is at the level of the stoma.

Paranasal Sinuses 5

Anatomy

Adjacent to the nasal cavity, are the paranasal cavities: maxillary, frontal, ethmoidal and sphenoidal. The ethmoid labyrinth is adjacent to the anterior cranial fossa. The lateral wall of the ethmoid is the medial wall of the orbit while the medial wall of the ethmoid sinus forms the lateral wall of the nose and attachment for the middle turbinate. Due to its close proximity to the nasal cavity, the ethmoid sinus is often involved when tumour extends from the nose into adjacent structures.

The maxillary sinus is the largest of the sinuses and encompasses the majority of the body of the maxilla. The walls of the maxillary sinus abutting the nasal cavity and orbit are thin whereas the anterior and posterior walls are relatively thick. The apices of the premolars and molars of the maxilla protrude into the maxillary sinus and are covered by a thin plate of bone. As the other sinuses do not form part of surgical resections in this area, they will not be discussed further.

Specimen

Specimens submitted for assessment of a maxillary tumour, mostly squamous cell cancer or a salivary gland tumour, usually consist of a hemimaxillectomy (Fig. 5.1, *page 96*). In the case of tumours situated in the roof of the maxillary sinus the palatal part of the maxilla may be left in situ (Figs. 5.2, 5.3, *page 97*). If there is tumour involvement of the orbital floor an orbital exenteration usually forms part of the specimen. In most instances the specimen is either a

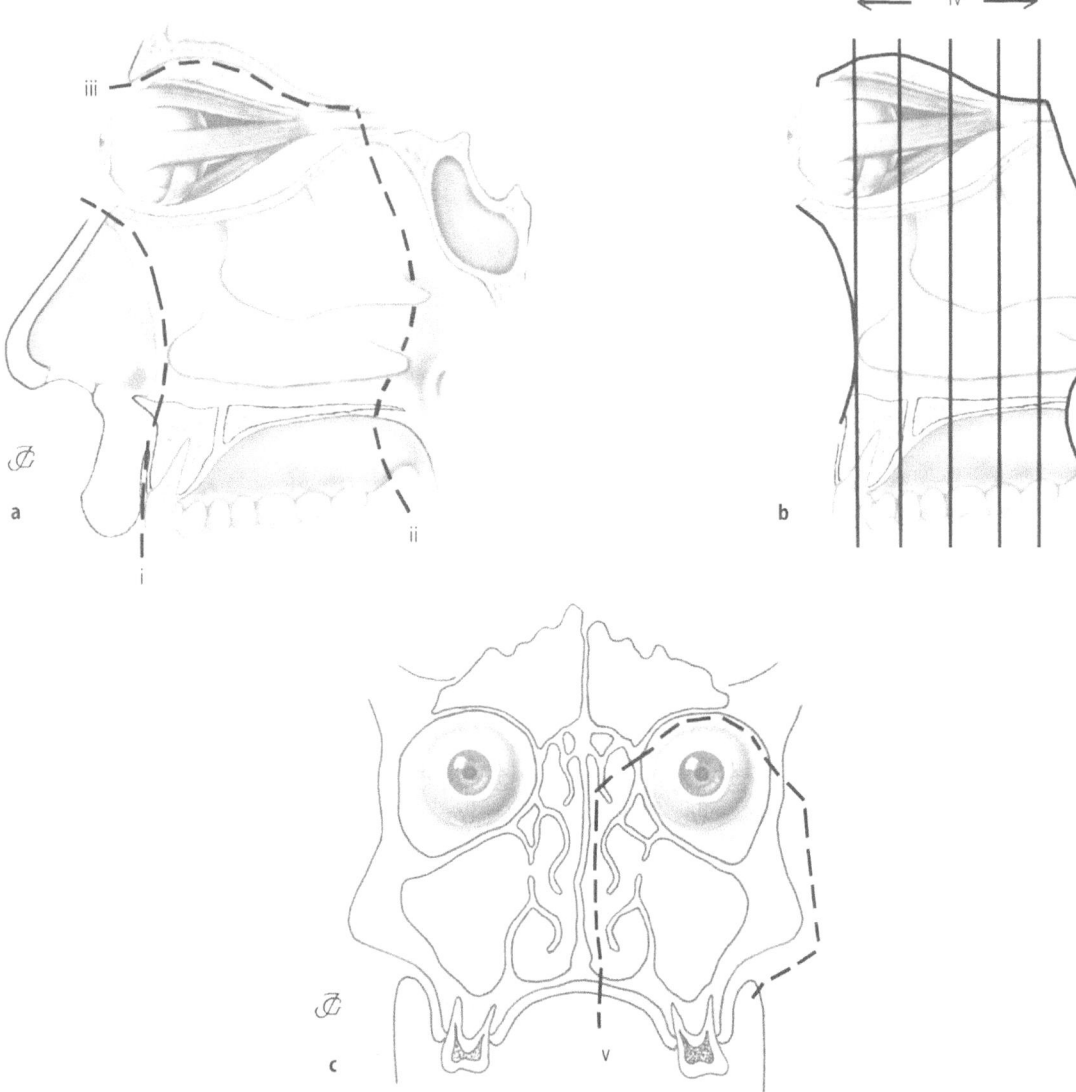

Figure 5.1
▲
Pathological anatomy of the maxillofacial complex.

a Medial view showing the lateral nasal wall with turbinates and the relationship of the nasal cavity with the orbit. Surgical margins of a hemimaxillectomy specimen with orbital exenteration are indicated by the dashed lines i–iii.

b Medial view of a hemimaxillectomy specimen with plane of sectioning iv parallel to the frontal plane.

c Frontal view showing the outline of a hemimaxillectomy with orbital exenteration. The medial vertical border v may be at either side of the nasal septum depending on the tumour site and location.

Figure 5.3
▶
a Macroscopic appearance of an orbital exenteration to treat tumour located in the roof of the maxillary sinus.

b Slice from the specimen showing the contents of the orbit as well as tumour present in the orbital floor and the orbital fatty tissue.

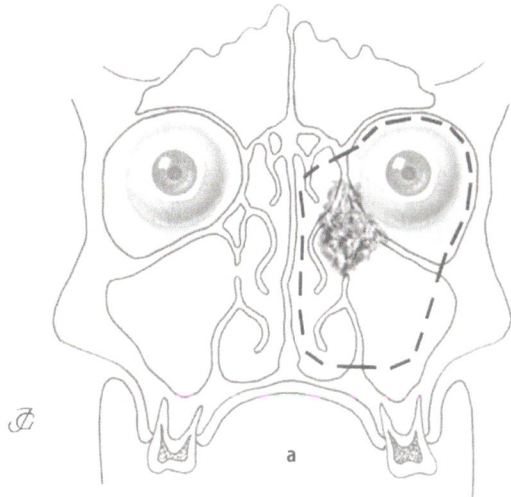 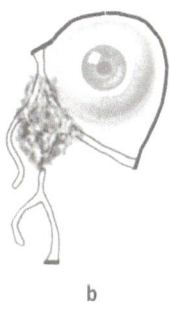

Pathological anatomy of a tumour in the roof of the maxillary sinus.

a Tumour shown in frontal projection together with outline of the resection.

b Cut surface when making slices as shown in Fig. 5.1, line iv. In these instances the orbital contents cannot be saved.

Figure 5.2
▲

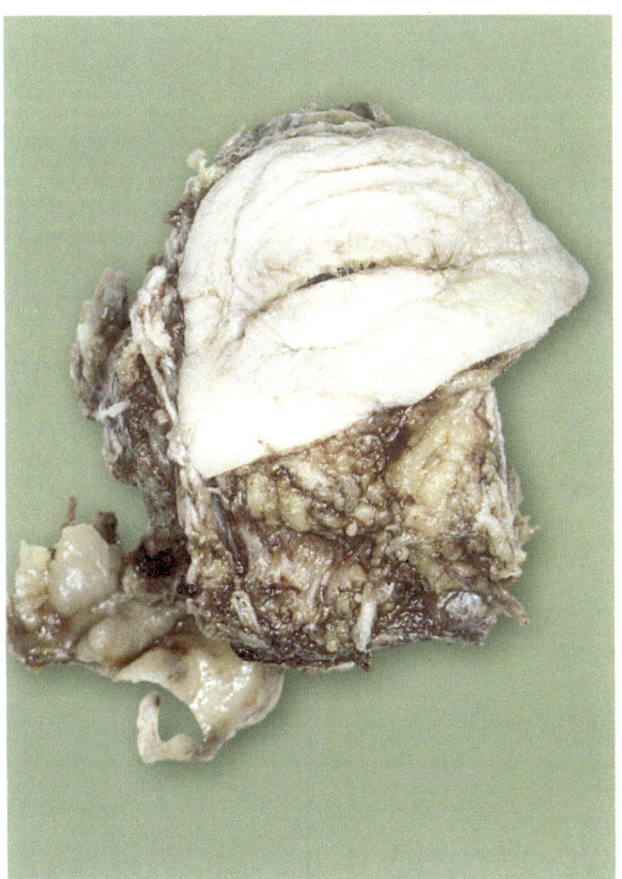 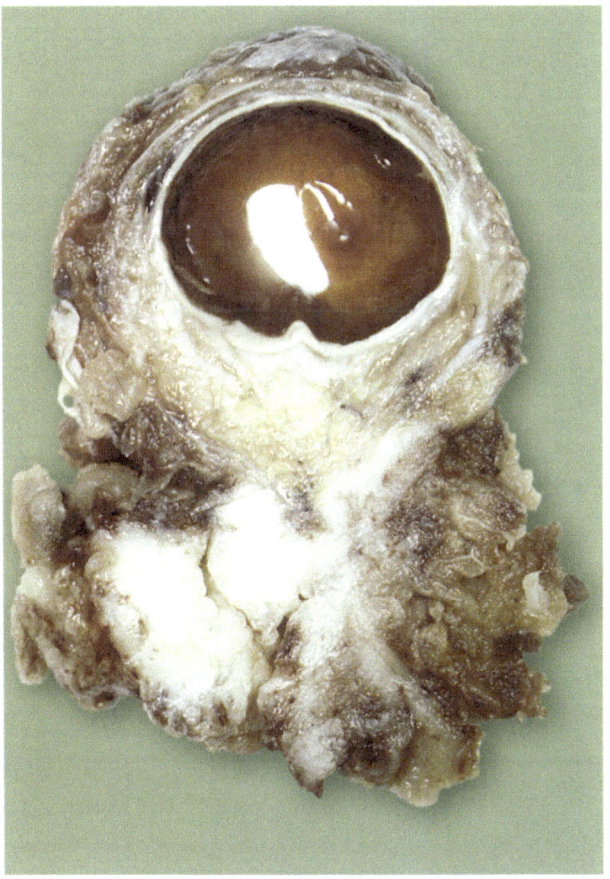

a   b

Figure 5.3

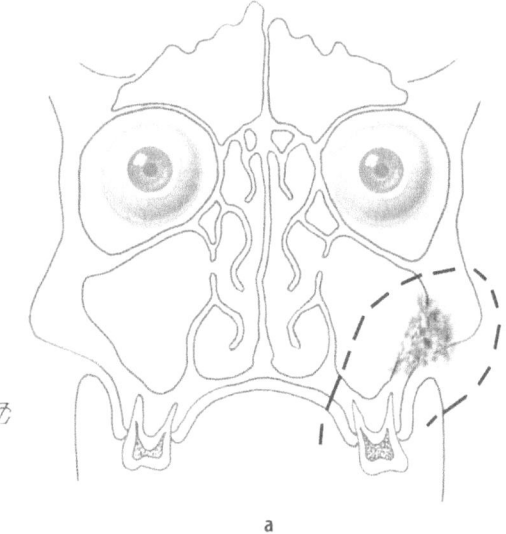
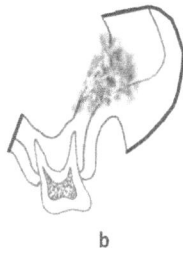

Figure 5.4
▲

Pathological anatomy of tumour in the bottom and lateral wall of the maxillary sinus.

a Tumour shown in frontal projection together with the outline of the resection.

b Cut surface when making slices as shown in Fig. 5.1, line iv. In these instances the orbital contents can be saved.

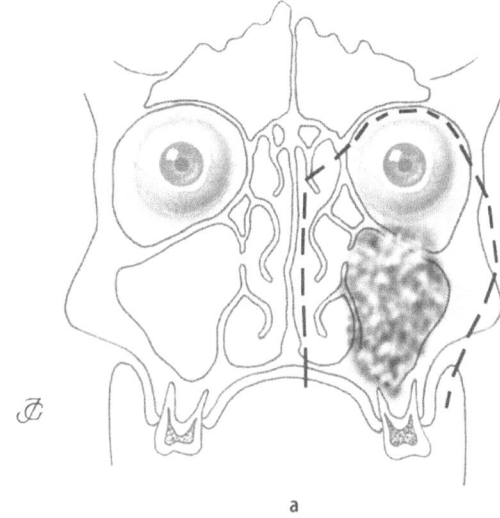
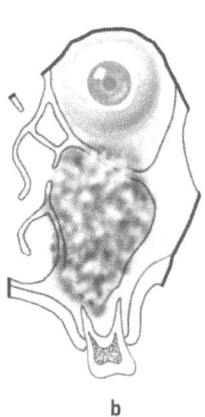

Figure 5.5
▲

Pathological anatomy of tumour occupying the entire maxillary sinus.

a Tumour shown in frontal projection together with outline of the resection.

b Cut surface when making slices as shown in Fig. 5.1, line iv. In these instances the orbital contents cannot be saved.

hemimaxillectomy (Fig. 5.4) or a hemimaxillectomy in continuity with an orbital exenteration.

Dissection

Investigation of the maxillectomy part of the specimen is done as outlined in the discussion on analysis of specimens removed for tumours of the maxilla in Chapter 2 (pp. 7–26). The specimen is sectioned parallel to the frontal plane and thus perpendicular to the palatal bone as well as the orbital floor. These slices also contain pieces of the eye globe if the contents of the orbit form part of the specimen. The slices allow assessment of the site of the tumour in the maxillary antrum, determination of whether there is destruction of the bony walls and analysis of spread in adjacent soft tissues (Figs. 5.5, *page 98*, 5.6, *page 100*). One should not forget to sample the contents of the pterygopalatine space for assessment of tumour spread in this area.

Specific attention should also be paid to the status of the orbital floor. Preoperatively there is often much discussion of whether and how the tumour involves this bony structure, and careful analysis of this bone plate will allow evaluation of pre-diagnostic imaging.

Surgical margins through these specimens are the same as for hemimaxillectomies proper, to which the margins through the ethmoid sinuses medial to the eye globe and the fatty tissue dorsal to the eye globe have to be added. One should also not forget to sample the optic nerve as well as the infraorbital nerve for analysis of perineural tumour spread.

Specific Features

Tumour may spread dorsally from the maxillary sinus into the pterygoid area or laterally through the bony wall into the infratemporal fossa. For assessment of margins in the case of spread dorsally into the pterygoid area, the dorsal part of the specimen has to be sliced horizontally; for assessment of spread into the infratemporal fossa, the usual slices parallel to the frontal plane are adequate to assess the tumour margins in this area (Fig. 5.7, *page 101*).

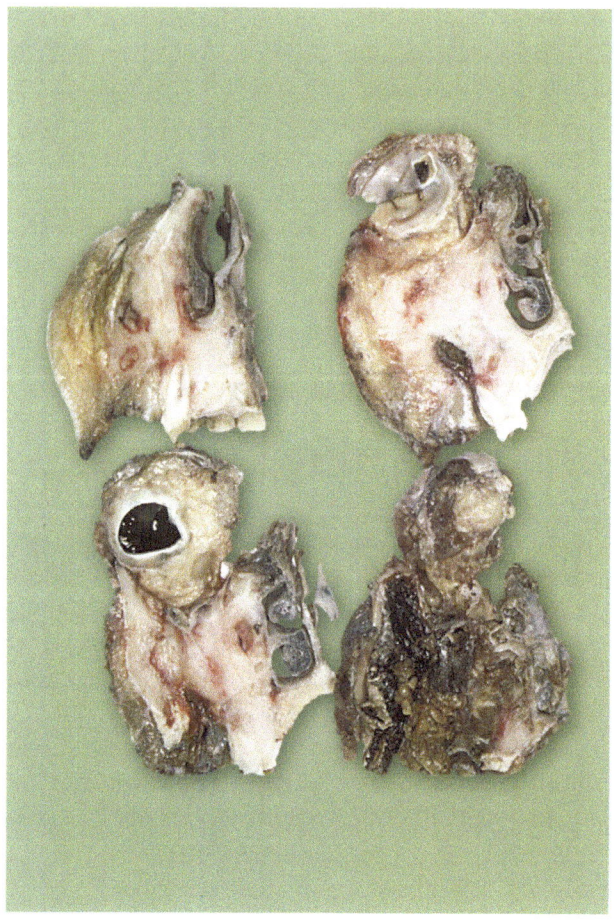

a

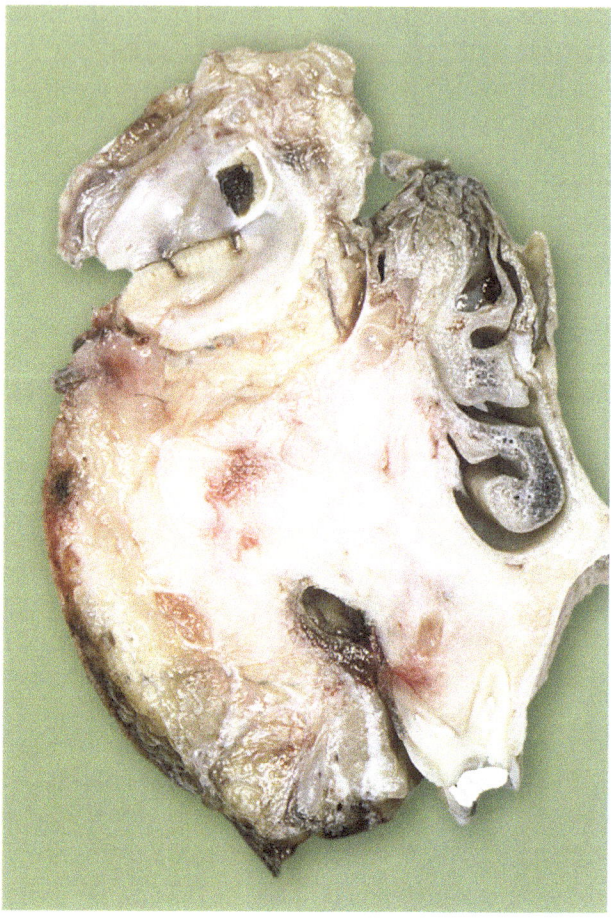

b

Figure 5.6

a Frontal slices from a hemimaxillectomy specimen with orbital exenteration to treat a maxillary leiomyosarcoma.

b A more detailed view of one of these slices shows tumour obliterating the maxillary sinus, spreading into the soft tissues of the cheek laterally, cranially destroying the orbital floor, and medially destroying the maxillary bone.

Figure 5.7

Pathological anatomy of tumour in the dorsal part of the maxillary sinus.

a Medial view through an opening in the partially removed lateral nasal wall into the maxillary sinus. Line i defines a plane shown in detail in **b**. Line ii defines a plane shown in detail in **d**.

b Horizontal projection to show extension of maxillary tumour into the infratemporal fossa or pterygoid area.

c Lateral view to show penetration of a maxillary sinus tumour through the lateral sinus wall. Lines i and ii define the planes mentioned in **a**.

d Frontal cut surface shows cranial extension of tumour into the infratemporal fossa.

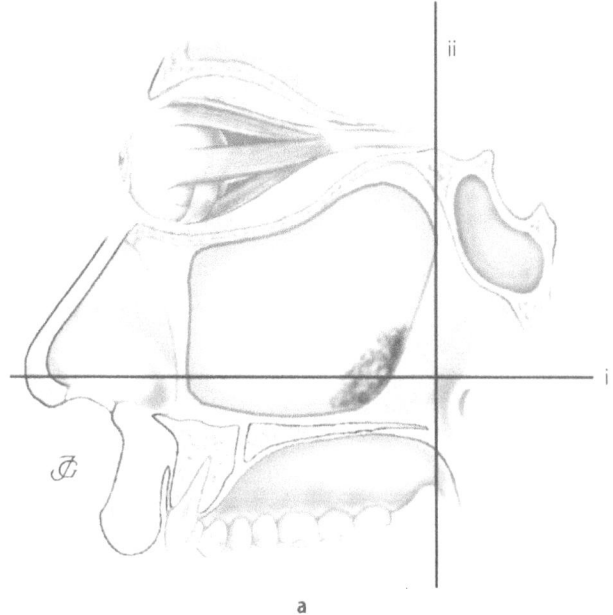

a

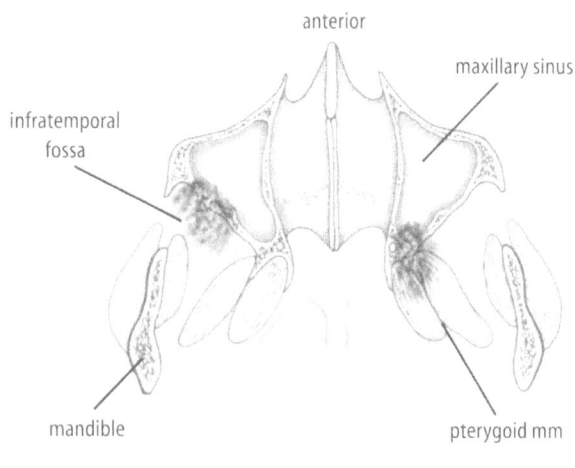

b

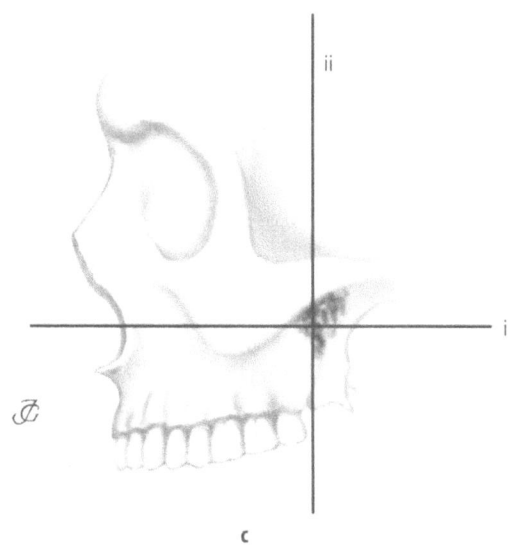

c

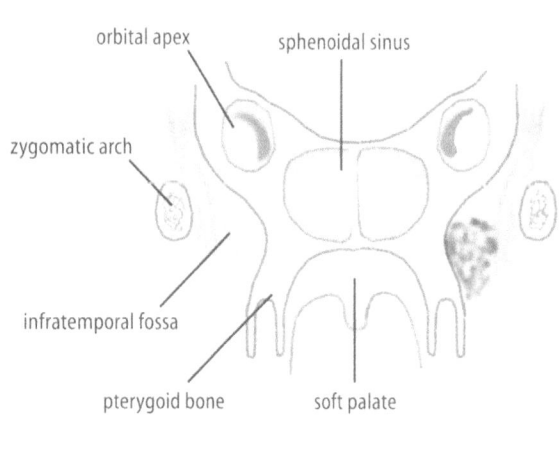

d

Figure 5.7

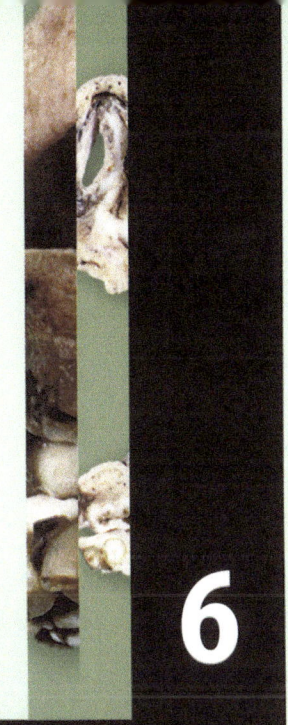

External Nose

6

Anatomy

The nasal cavity has a roof, floor, lateral wall and septum. Its anterior part is the nasal vestibule that is bordered inferiorly by the palatine process of the maxilla, medially by the septum cartilage, and laterally as well as superiorly by the soft tissues of the external nose.

Specimen

Removal of the external nose is usually done for treatment of squamous cell cancer of the nasal vestibule. If the tumour lies anteriorly the specimen may consist of only the nose itself. If the tumour lies more dorsally the specimen may contain parts of the soft tissues of the upper lip and of the anterior maxillary bone, as removal of parts of these adjacent areas may be required to obtain tumour-free margins.

Dissection

Analysis of the specimen starts with inspection and recording which structures form part of it. The site of the tumour should be noted as well as its size. Thereafter the specimen is cut in parallel slices. The plane of sectioning usually lies parallel to the dorsal surface of the specimen. This dorsal surface contains three surgical margins: two through right and left nasal wings and one through the median nasal septum. In making these slices, marks are needed to identify right and left sides to avoid confusion about which side contains tumour when

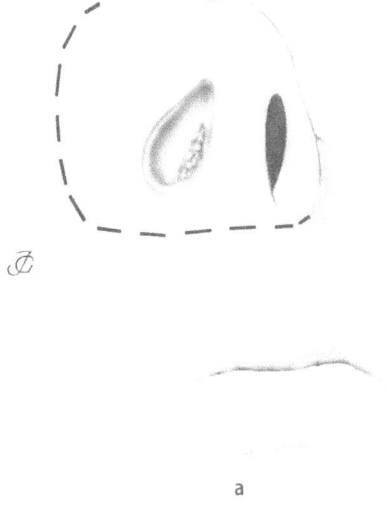

a

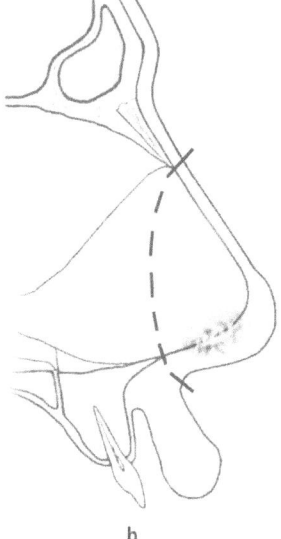

b

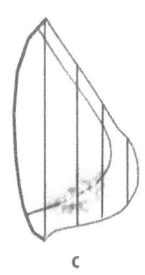

c

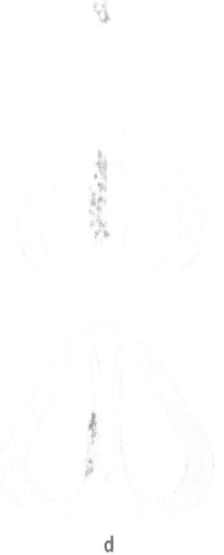

d

Figure 6.1	Pathological anatomy of cancer of the nasal vestibule.

▲

a Clinical appearance of tumour and outline of the resection.

b Sagittal view to show the relationship of tumour with its surroundings and outline of the resection.

c Sagittal view of the surgical specimen removed, conforming to the dashed outlines in **a** and **b**. Vertical lines indicate levels of sectioning.

d Slices obtained when cutting the specimen according to the levels shown in **c**.

examining the histological sections. The slices thus obtained allow visualisation of tumour thickness, depth of penetration and spread into adjacent structures, e.g. from one nasal cavity to the other by perforation of the nasal septum. For specimens consisting only of the external nose without adjacent structures, this approach is adequate (Figs. 6.1, page 104, 6.2, page 106).

Analysis of specimens containing parts of the anterior maxilla or the upper lip is far more complicated. These specimens have multiple surgical margins lying in different planes and in these cases parallel sectioning will not yield adequate information about these margins. It is therefore necessary to sample margins before slicing the nasal part of the specimen parallel to the dorsal surface. In the case of specimens containing nose as well as upper lip, one has to assess whether the lip excision extends into the free margin of the upper lip or whether the surgeon has performed a partial lip excision while saving the free margin including the vermilion border. In the case of a full-thickness lip removal one starts by sampling right and left lip margins, similar to the approach for wedge excisions of lip specimens, which is done by cutting vertical slices perpendicular to the vermilion border. If the lower part of the upper lip is saved one has to evaluate the horizontal surgical margin through the lip, which is done by making a slice parallel to this surgical margin. Thereafter the specimen can be sliced according to the guidelines for specimens of the nose proper, the more ventral slices going through the lip. In the case of specimens containing the anterior part of the maxillary bone, dissection can be done in the usual way by cutting slices parallel to the dorsal surgical margin. These slices will be lengthened caudally to include the maxillary bone. Both lateral margins as well as the dorsal margin through the maxillary bone are clearly displayed in this way, allowing evaluation of tumour spread in this area. For nose specimens containing parts of lip as well as maxillary bone the combined guidelines apply (Figs. 6.3, page 107, 6.4, page 108).

Specific Features

Quite often nose excisions are done for tumour that recurs after irradiation. In these instances the macroscopic features are difficult to evaluate as fibrosis and tumour are not easily discernible with the naked eye. One should therefore sample more extensively for histological examination.

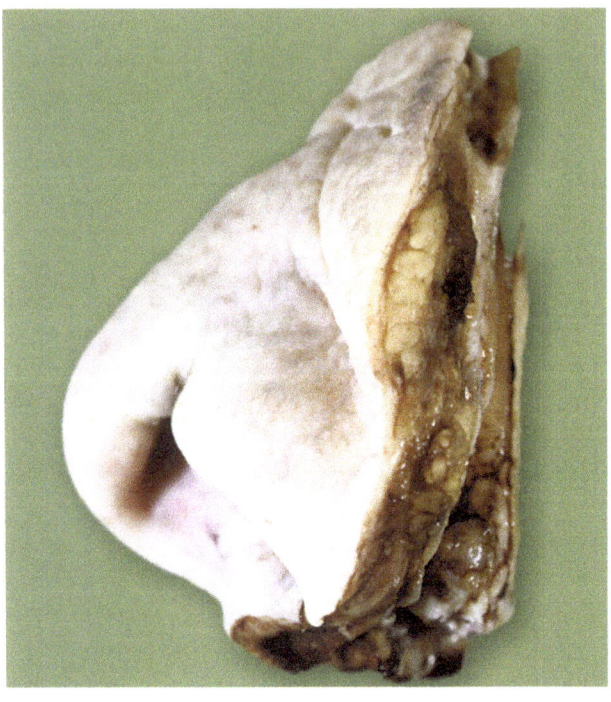

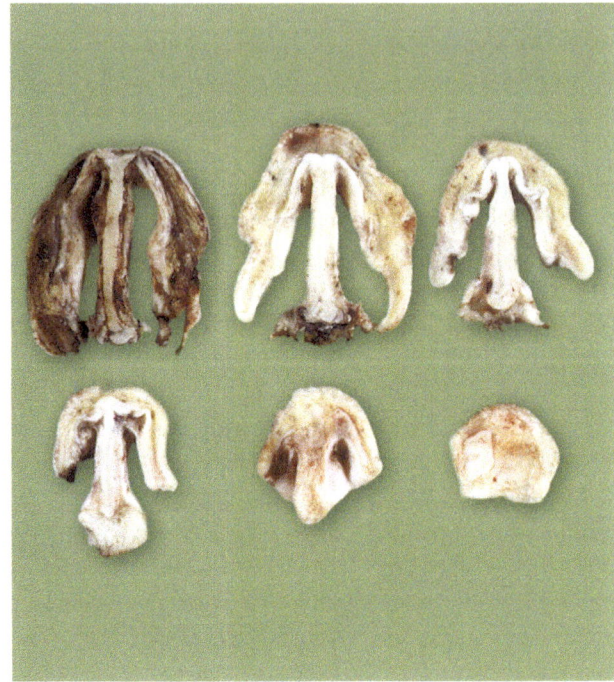

a

b

Figure 6.2 ▲

a Macroscopic appearance of nose amputation due to cancer of the nasal vestibule. Lateral view.

b Horizontal slices showing tumour extension.

Figure 6.3 ▶

Pathological anatomy of cancer of the nasal vestibule extending into the upper lip and/or anterior part of the maxilla.

a Extension of resection through the facial skin. In this instance the upper lip is partly saved. These resections may also contain the entire median part of the upper lip including the vermilion border.

b Extension of resection through the anterior maxilla.

c Sagittal view of tumour and extension into adjacent areas. Dashed lines i and ii indicate surgical margins. In the case of full-thickness lip resections there is only a dorsal surgical margin as indicated by line i.

d Sagittal view of surgical specimen with levels of sectioning parallel to the dorsal surface. Previously the horizontal resection margin through the lip that lies in a different plane has been sampled as indicated by line iii. When the specimen contains the complete median part of the upper lip including the vermilion border there is no horizontal surgical margin through the lip, this part of the specimen including the free edge of the upper lip.

e Anterior view of the surgical specimen to illustrate the sampling of the resection margins through the upper lip that are in different planes. Samples are taken from right and left vertical margins through the upper lip and a sample is taken horizontally between the cranial part of the upper lip that forms part of the specimen and the caudal part including the vermilion border that is left in situ. If the specimen contains the caudal part of the lip and the vermilion border as well, then only left and right vertical margins have to be sampled before slicing the specimen parallel to the dorsal surface as shown in **d**.

f Sections obtained by slicing from dorsal to ventral as shown in **d**. Note that anteriorly the specimen has fallen apart into two separate structures: the anterior maxillary alveolar process with the teeth and the external nose with the adherent part of the upper lip. The most ventral slice goes through the tip of the nose and does not contain any surgical margins.

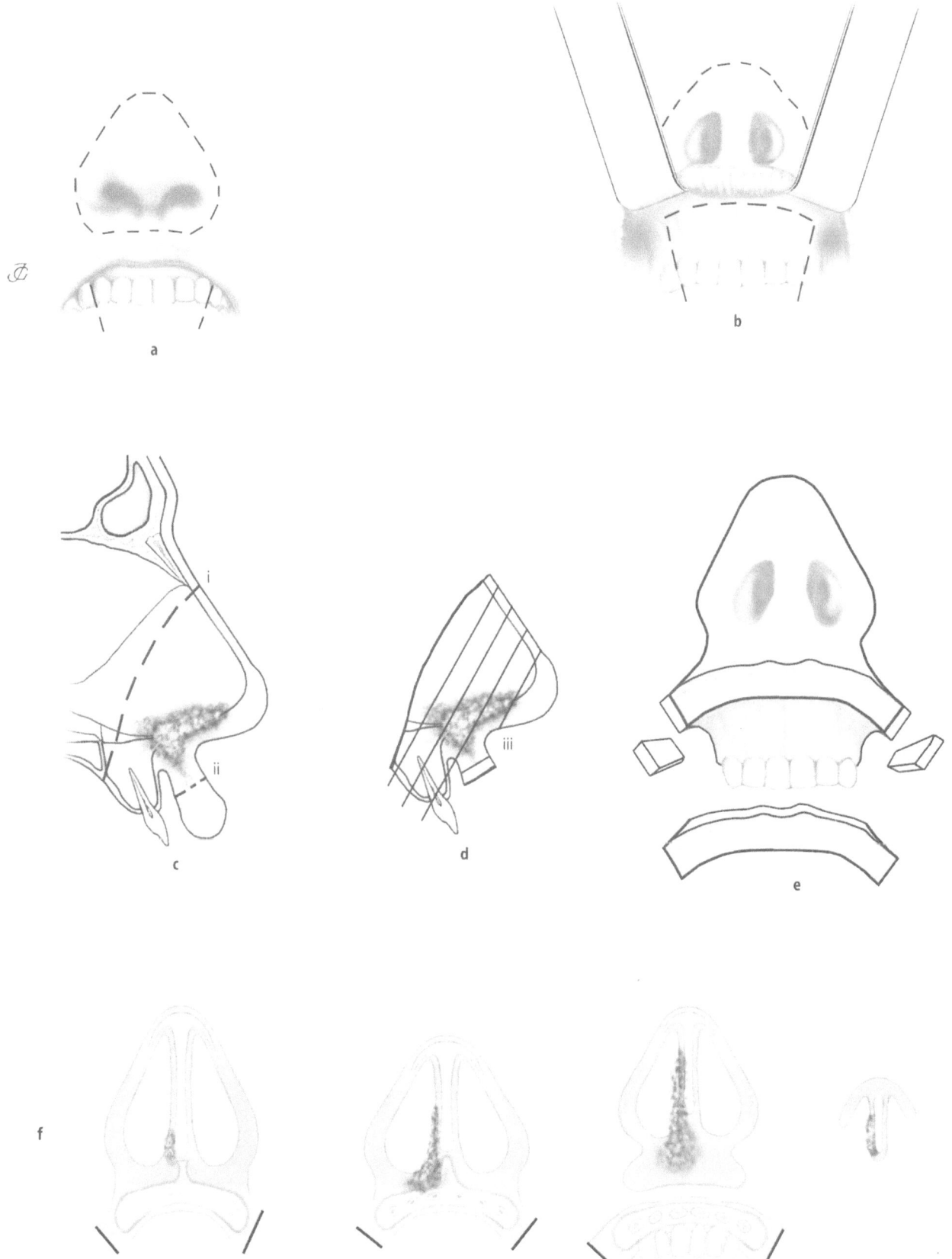

Figure 6.3

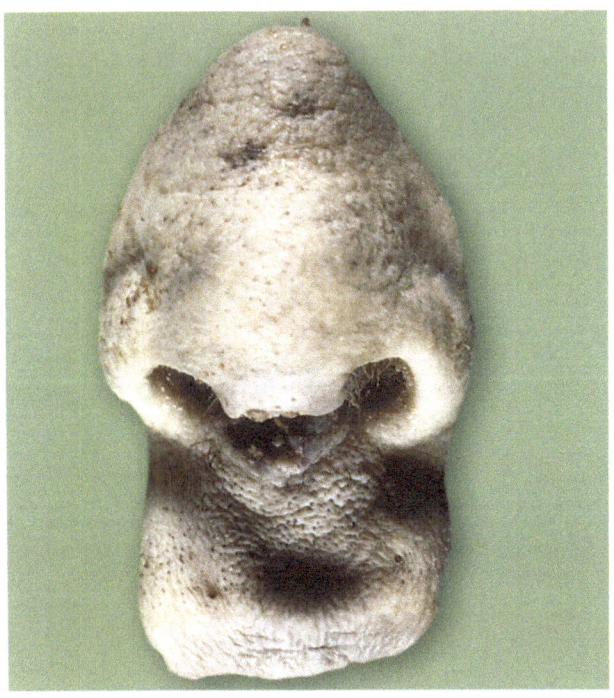

a

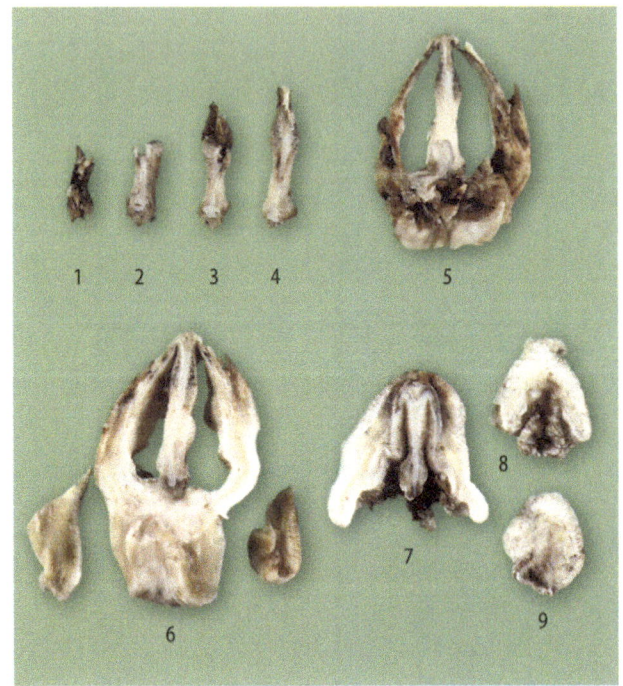

b

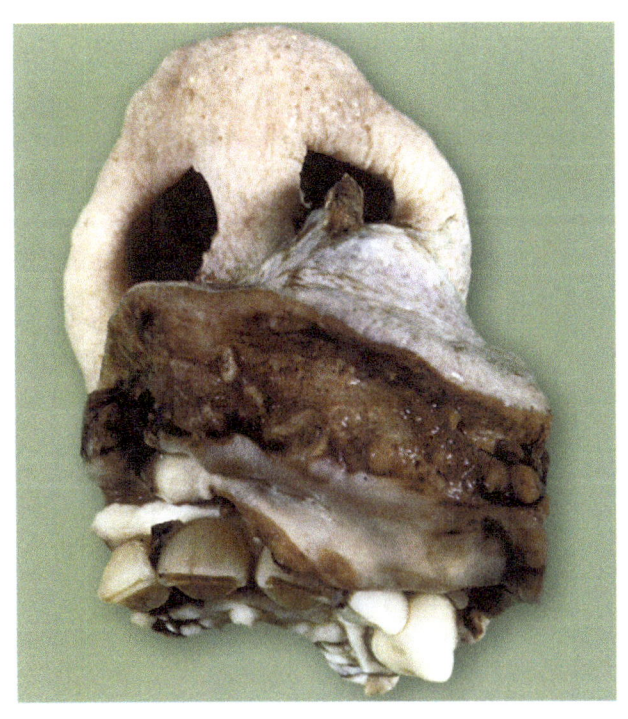

c

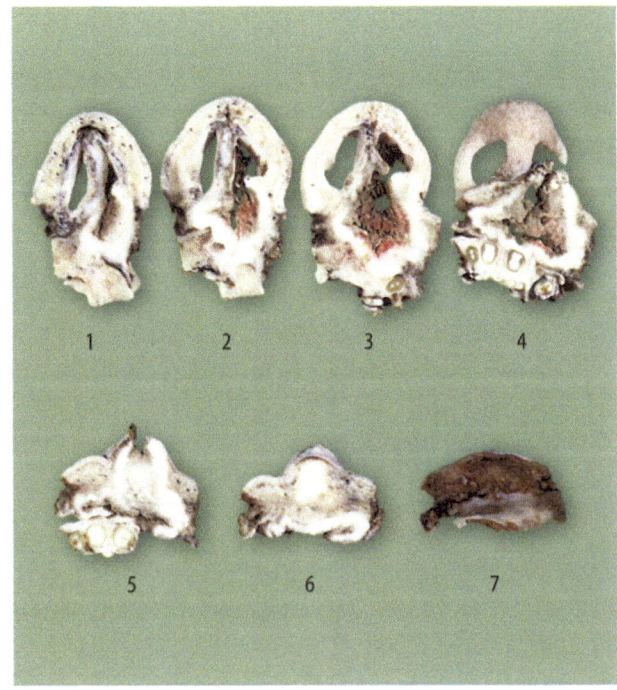

d

Figure 6.4

Macroscopic appearances of external nose resections including the lip and/or anterior maxilla.

a Anterior view of specimen containing the nose as well as the complete median part of the upper lip.

b Slices obtained by cutting the specimen parallel to the dorsal surface. Slices 1–4 contain only the nasal septum, which sometimes protrudes dorsally beyond the level of resection margins through right and left wings. Slice 5 is the first complete slice containing the septum as well as both wings. Slice 6 goes through the upper lip; right and left labial margins are sampled separately and these are the two separate tissue fragments lying adjacent to the lip part of this slice. Slices 7–9 are through the tip of the nose and do not contain surgical margins.

c Anterior view of specimen containing the nose as well as the anterior maxilla with teeth and part of the upper lip. In this case the lower part of the upper lip including the vermilion border is not included in the resection.

d Slices 1–7 are cut from dorsally to ventrally. In slice 5 the maxillary part has become separate from the nasal part of the specimen. Slices 6 and 7 contain only the lip part of the specimen.

Figure 6.4
◄

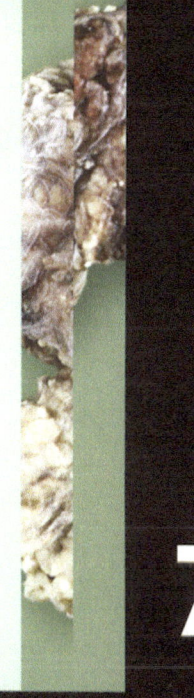

Neck Dissections

7

Anatomy

A neck dissection consists of a tissue mass containing the cervical lymphatics. In its classical form it extends from the submandibular soft tissues to the supraclavicular fatty tissue, bordered laterally by platysma and medially by the internal jugular vein (Fig. 7.1, *page 112*). Historically the lymph nodes in this area are divided into six compartments, the so-called levels. In describing these levels we will use the terminology adopted by the American Academy of Otolaryngology's Committee for Head and Neck Surgery and Oncology [3] (Fig. 7.2, *page 113*).

Level I is subdivided into two compartments: the submental area that lies between both anterior bellies of the digastric muscle and the hyoid bone dorsally, and the submandibular area that lies between the anterior belly of the digastric muscle medially and the mandibular bone laterally. Dorsally this area is bordered by the tendon between anterior and posterior belly of the digastric muscle, which is attached to the hyoid bone, and the posterior belly of the digastric muscle itself. Thus the triangle of soft tissue enclosed anteriorly and laterally by the mandible and dorsally by the hyoid is subdivided into one median compartment (the submental area) and two lateral compartments (the submandibular areas).

Level II represents the upper jugular (cervical) group of lymph nodes. This area extends from the base of the skull superiorly to the carotid bifurcation or hyoid bone inferiorly. The nodes in this area mainly cluster in the vicinity of the internal jugular vein and are laterally covered by the body of the sternocleidomastoid muscle.

Level III represents the middle jugular (cervical) group of lymph nodes. These nodes are located around the middle third of the internal jugular vein

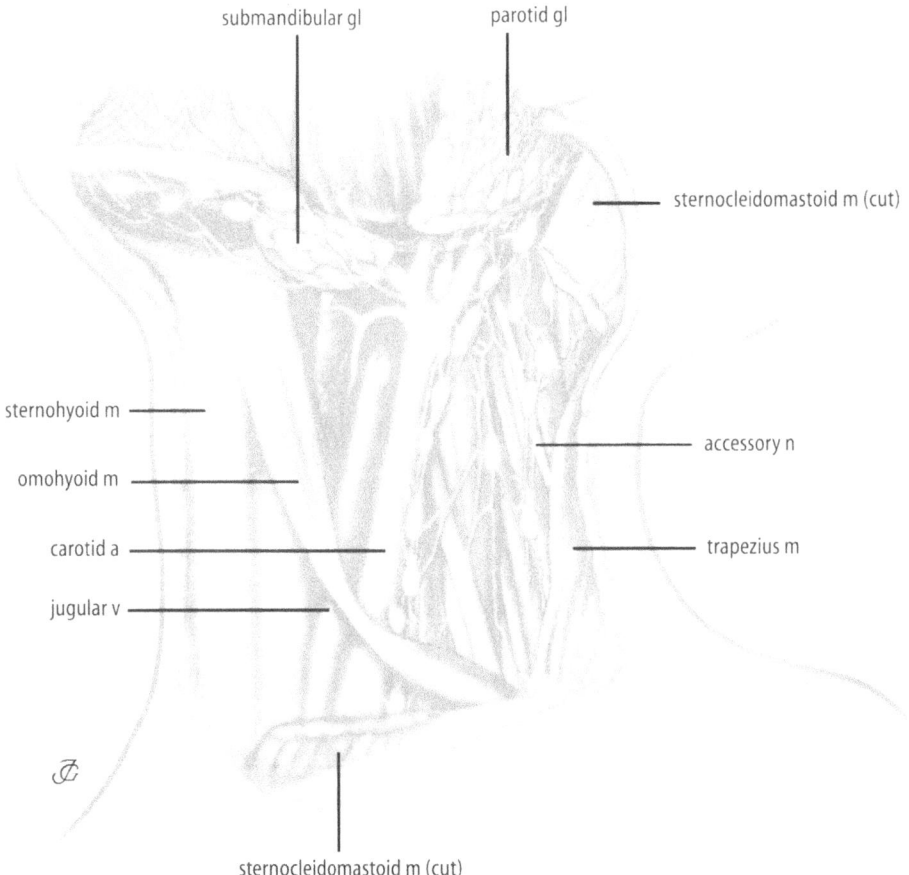

submandibular gl   parotid gl

sternocleidomastoid m (cut)

sternohyoid m

omohyoid m

carotid a

jugular v

accessory n

trapezius m

sternocleidomastoid m (cut)

Figure 7.1   Surgical anatomy of neck dissection. Important structures are labelled.

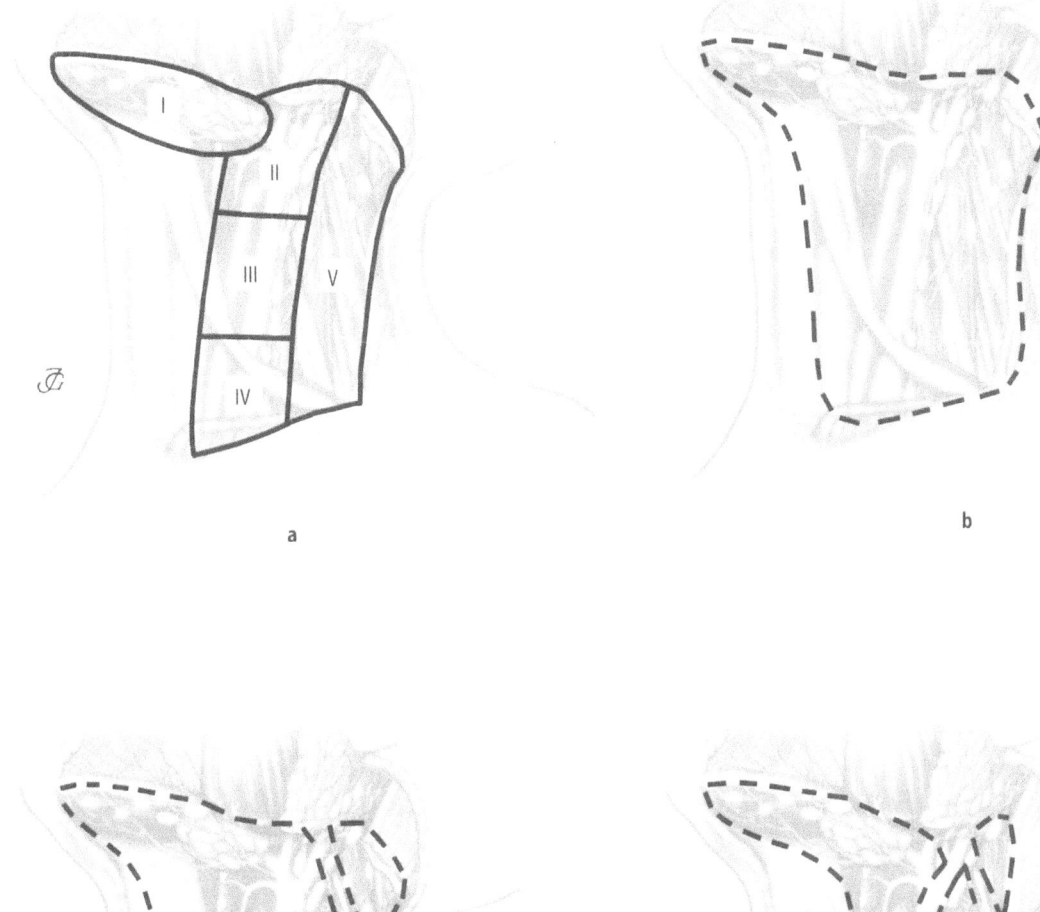

Pathological anatomy of neck dissection.

a Lymph node levels projected onto the neck tissues.

b Outline of radical neck dissection.

c Outline of modified radical neck dissection in which the accessory nerve is saved.

d Outline of supraomohyoid neck dissection that includes nodes from levels I–III while leaving non-lymphatic tissues in situ.

Figure 7.2
▲

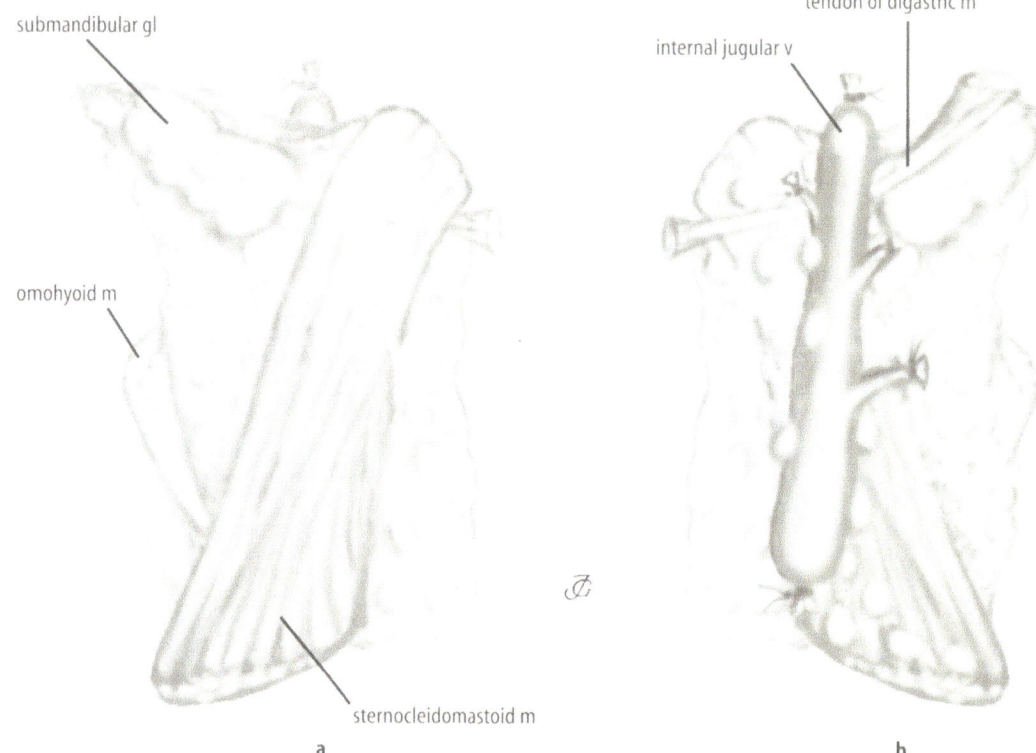

submandibular gl

omohyoid m

sternocleidomastoid m

a

internal jugular v

tendon of digastric m

b

Figure 7.3
▲

Pathological anatomy of a radical neck dissection specimen.

a Lateral view showing the submandibular gland, omohyoid muscle and sternocleidomastoid muscle.

b Medial view showing the submandibular gland, internal jugular vein and digastric tendon that is the anatomical landmark allowing distinction between nodes from level I and level II.

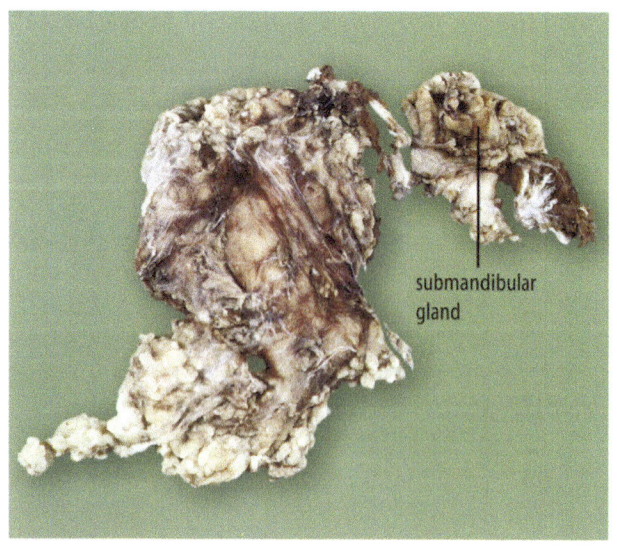

submandibular gland

a

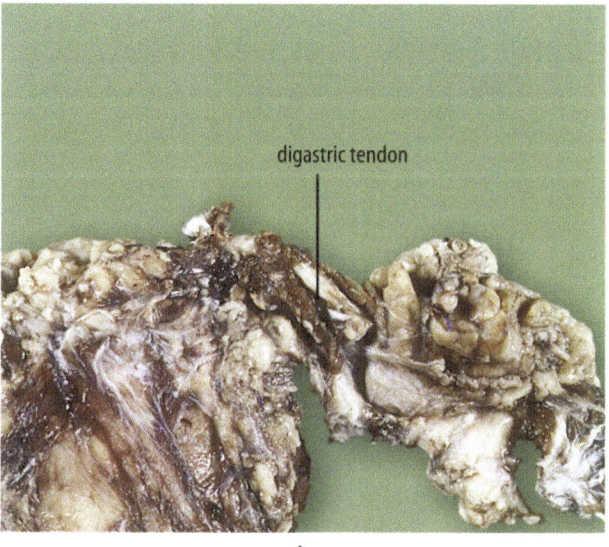

digastric tendon

b

Figure 7.4

that begins superiorly where the upper jugular compartment ends; the lower border lies at the level of the cricothyroid notch.

Level IV comprises the lymph nodes located around the lower third of the internal jugular vein, extending from the omohyoid muscle superiorly to the clavicle inferiorly.

Level V comprises the nodes that collectively form the posterior triangle group. This is a triangular area lying between the anterior border of the trapezius muscle posteriorly, the posterior border of the sternocleidomastoid muscle anteriorly and the clavicle caudally. This level includes the supraclavicular nodes.

Level VI is the anterior compartment. This compartment has the hyoid as its cranial and the suprasternal notch as its caudal border. Both lateral borders are the medial boundaries of the carotid sheath. This area is thus a rectangle that lies between the area defined as level I above and the sternum below.

Specimen

There are two main reasons for performing a neck dissection. The first indication is to remove metastatic deposits in the neck nodes that have been diagnosed by time-honoured clinical methods such as inspection and palpation or by more sophisticated methods such as ultrasound-guided fine needle aspiration. In that case the patient is classified as N+.

A neck dissection will also be performed if the patient suffers from a tumour with a high risk for neck node metastasis. Although objective evidence for neck node metastasis is not found, a neck dissection will nevertheless be done for preventive reasons. This is mainly the case with squamous cell cancers of the mobile tongue and floor of the mouth, oropharynx and hypopharynx.

Neck dissection specimens may be of varying nature. In the past a variety of surgical procedures

has led to a plethora of terms, but thanks to the efforts of the American Academy of Otolaryngology's Committee [3] the current classification recognises only four different types that we will discuss now, using the above-defined levels as a guideline (Fig. 7.2, page 113).

A radical neck dissection consists of the nodes from level I to level V. The internal jugular vein, sternocleidomastoid muscle and spinal accessory nerve also form part of it. If only the lymphatic structures are removed this is termed a modified radical neck dissection. The non-lymphatic structures that may be left in situ could be the internal jugular vein, the sternocleidomastoid muscle or the spinal accessory nerve. The structures thus saved should be specifically mentioned by the surgeon when submitting such a specimen to the pathology laboratory.

If less than levels I–V is removed the neck dissection is termed selective. Four different types of selective neck dissection are recognised. In the case of a supraomohyoid neck dissection, nodes from levels I to III are removed. A posterolateral neck dissection comprises levels II–V as well as nodes located suboccipitally and lying retroauricularly that are not contained within levels I–VI. A lateral neck dissection refers to removal of the nodes from levels II to IV. In the case of an anterior compartment neck dissection the nodes from level VI are removed.

Extended radical neck dissection is the fourth type. This term refers to any type of neck dissection that consists of a radical neck dissection together with additional structures, either lymphatic or non-lymphatic, that have to be identified specifically. These structures may be additional lymph node compartments, nerves or blood vessels.

In head and neck surgical pathology the neck dissections most often encountered are the radical neck dissection, the modified radical neck dissection and the supraomohyoid neck dissection. The other types of neck dissections are done for lesions outside the upper aerodigestive tract, e.g.

a Medial view of a specimen from a radical neck dissection.

b Detailed view from the upper part of a radical neck dissection specimen to show the digastric tendon that forms the border between the submandibular and upper jugular nodes.

Figure 7.4
◄

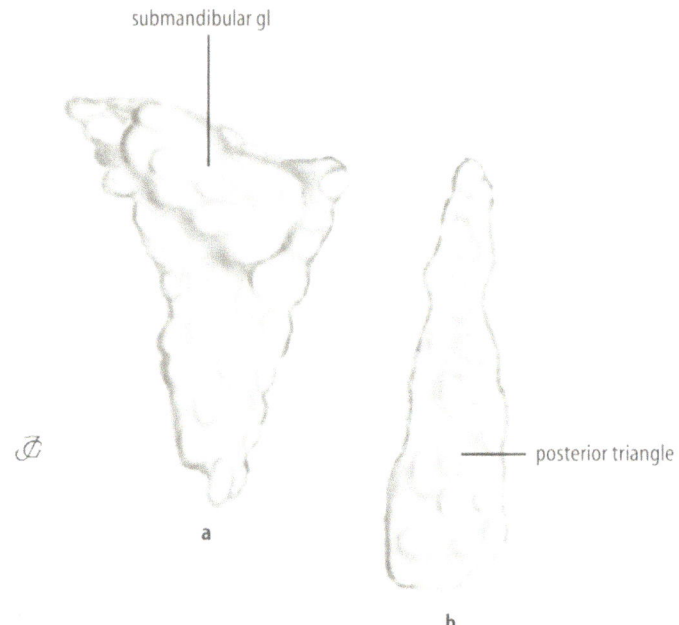

submandibular gl

posterior triangle

a

b

Figure 7.5
▲

a, b Pathological anatomy of a supraomohyoid neck dissection specimen. The submandibular gland defines the cranial part of the specimen.

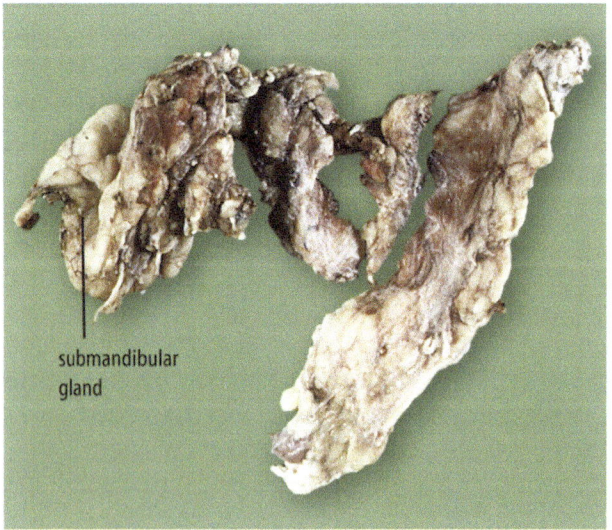

submandibular
gland

Figure 7.6
▲

Macroscopic appearance of a supraomohyoid neck dissection specimen. Only the submandibular gland can be recognised as an anatomical landmark.

for malignancies of the scalp or thyroid gland. Therefore we will only discuss the examination of radical, modified radical and supraomohyoid dissections.

Dissection

Examination of a neck dissection should be done with the following questions in mind: (1) Does the specimen contain lymph nodes with metastatic deposits? (2) If it does, how many lymph nodes with metastasis are present, specified for each level? (3) Is there gross extracapsular tumour spread?

Dissection of the specimen starts with determination of the type of neck dissection and identification of the several levels that form part of it. As the anatomical boundaries that are used by surgeons to identify the levels are not all present within the specimen, these cannot be used by the pathologist. Therefore another approach is needed, which will be discussed for each type of neck dissection separately.

In the case of the prototypical specimen, the radical neck dissection, four different anatomical landmarks have to be identified: the submandibular gland, the tendon between the posterior and anterior belly of the digastric muscle, the sternocleidomastoid muscle and the internal jugular vein (Figs. 7.3, 7.4, page 114). Recognition of the submandibular gland enables identification of the ventrocranial side of the specimen and, together with surrounding fatty tissue, forms level I. The digastric tendon forms the boundary between level I and level II. The internal jugular vein lies medially to the sternocleidomastoid muscle; it enables identification of levels II, III and IV by division into three equal parts from cranial to caudal. Level V lies dorsal to the caudal half of the sternocleidomastoid muscle. To facilitate this examination it may be helpful to imagine the radical neck dissection as a capital Z, its upper horizontal line representing level I, its lower horizontal line being level V, and levels II, III and IV forming three equal parts of the oblique connecting line.

In the case of a modified radical neck dissection, identification of the levels comprising the specimen may be more complicated if the surgeon has not indicated the boundaries by using coloured beads or other markings. Level I can still be recognised by its association with the submandibular gland, but the other levels in this type of neck dissection consist merely of a mass of fatty tissue without anatomical landmarks that can be roughly divided into cranial, caudal and dorsal but without further details.

In the case of a supraomohyoid neck dissection, again the submandibular gland allows identification of level I, while levels II and III can be defined by dividing the fatty tissue mass dorsal to the submandibular gland into two equal halves, the cranial half being level II and the caudal half being level III. The upper border of level II sometimes contains a small portion of the caudal part of the parotid gland that facilitates determination of which part of the fatty tissue dorsal to the submandibular gland is cranial and which caudal (Figs. 7.5, 7.6).

After this first inspection one should record whether there are any externally visible enlarged lymph nodes and, if there are, which level they form a part of. These nodes should be measured, removed from the specimen and sampled for histological examination; it is wise to ink their outer surface beforehand to allow evaluation of extracapsular spread into the surface of the specimen. Then, if present, the internal jugular vein should be opened and the blood clot in it removed. This enables inspection of the luminal surface for tumour spread across the venous wall. Thereafter the specimen should be cut into thin parallel slices: for levels I and V vertically and for levels II–IV horizontally. For levels II–V this sectioning should be done from medial to lateral, thus saving the most lateral part of the sternocleidomastoid muscle and in this way preserving the integrity of the specimen. By doing this all nodes from each level can be identified and sampled for histological examination. The macroscopic description of the specimen should include the number of nodes from each level, irrespective of their status. The size of the nodes should also be recorded. In the case of gross extracapsular tumour spread approaching the surface of the specimen, the outer surface of the slice with the minimum distance between tumour and surface should be inked to evaluate whether there is tumour growth into the surface in this area.

References

1. Association of Directors of Anatomic and Surgical Pathology (1997) Recommendations for the reporting of larynx specimens containing laryngeal neoplasms. Virchows Arch 431:155–157
2. Michaels L, Gregor RT (1980) Examination of the larynx in the histopathology laboratory. J Clin Pathol 33:705–710
3. Robbins KT, Medina JE, Wolfe GT, Levine PA, Sessions RB, Pruet CW (1991) Standardising neck dissection terminology. Official report of the Academy's committee for head and neck surgery and oncology. Arch Otolaryngol Head Neck Surg 117:601–605

Index

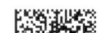